FOOD OF THE GODS

Morocco Gold
Extra Virgin Olive Oil

By

Gordon Davidson

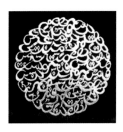

First published in the USA 2022 by Amazon

Gordon Davidson have asserted their right under the Copyright, Designs and Patents Act, 1988, to be identified as the Author of this work.

Cover image: Morocco Gold Ltd.

Amazon does not have any control over, or responsibility for, any third-party websites referred to or in this book. All internet addresses given in this book were correct at the time of going to press. The author and publishers regret any inconvenience caused if addresses have changed or sites have ceased to exist but can accept no responsibility for any such changes.

Every effort has been made to trace the copyright holders and obtain permission to reproduce copyright material, both illustrative and quoted. We apologise for any omissions in this respect and will be pleased to make appropriate acknowledgements in any future editions.

978-1-958324-66-0

www.morocco-gold.com

www.facebook.com/MoroccoGold

www.twitter.com/MoroccoGold

www.instagram.com/morocco.gold/

THANKS & ACKNOLEDGEMENTS

To all the wonderful people in Morocco who have welcomed us into their families and have helped to bring Morocco Gold to fruition.

FOREWORD

In an ever changing and fast-moving world, exponential rates of progress in understanding the universe and our place in it, unlocking the secrets of quantum physics, unravelling genetic codes and a myriad of new discoveries unlocked by scientific understanding, it is unusual to re-discover a 'wisdom of the ancients' that is as potent now as it has been for thousands of years.

At a time when national and cross-cultural tensions are rising it is also wonderful to create a cross cultural venture where people of 'good heart' can come together to create something that people from all different cultures and background can benefit from.

This is what makes the story of Morocco Gold extra virgin olive oil unique and fascinating

DISCLAIMER

Information included in this book reflects interpretation of current research evidence, based on peer reviewed publications in scientific literature involving population observational and controlled trials of adult populations. It should not replace the guidance of prescribed medication of a personal physician. In the event of allergies or special prescribed diets, further medical direction should be sought.

Reference to this information should be made in support of making positive changes in diet and lifestyle.

Regular exercise is also important to maintain a good state of health and wellbeing. If any individual has concerns about their need or capacity to make lifestyle changes, they should seek further medical advice.

.

CONTENTS

INTRODUCTION

Scotland is a wonderful country to live in. It has a wonderful heritage, outstanding natural beauty, and history that knocks Game Of Thrones into a cocked hat. When the sun shines, it is the most wonderful place on earth to be. Unfortunately, the sun does not shine in Scotland for much of the year.

My lifetime of work as a management consultant, transforming businesses and their performance, has, however, taken me to many parts of Europe and the USA where the sun does shine. This, together with the business challenges faced, great people I have had the privilege of working with, has made this an incredibly rewarding career in so many ways.

However, this was interrupted when my wife, soulmate, and best friend Linda, also a mainstay of our consultancy business, was diagnosed with breast cancer. This gave us an additional, life-changing project to manage. There was never any doubt that Linda would recover however this 2-year period prompted a re-evaluation of life's priorities.

We also decided we would look for our own 'place in the sun'. We looked around Europe, countries I had worked in, looked at the logistics of traveling between countries, then spotted an article about Morocco and its resurgence as a 'go-to' destination of choice. Being only a 4-hour flight from Edinburgh to Marrakech, we decided to explore and wow!

On the very first visit, we were captivated by the colours, sights, and exotic aromas of Marrakech, the sheer vibrancy of Marrakech, and the warmth and friendliness of its people. We decided quite quickly – this was the place for us. So, we renovated a Riad, a traditional house in the centre of the old medina in Marrakech, to be our 'place in the sun'. Some of our friends thought we were barking mad, however, but this is where my project management background from my consultancy days came to the fore, and the project was successfully completed on time and on budget. The story of our renovation is worth a book in itself. It also gave us a real insight into the workings and administrative challenges of living in Morocco. Linda now runs the Riad as a highly successful guest house business in Marrakech and is a key social media influencer in the city.

Whilst we were settling in, we also made a point of traveling extensively throughout the country to discover less well-known Morocco. From Tangier, where you can still feel the 'edginess' of a city that was once an international protectorate during World War II and full of spies watching each other, the green, rolling Rif mountains with its blue-washed mountain town of Chefchaouen, one of Morocco's most picturesque villages, the rich and fertile fields surrounding the agricultural centre of Meknes, nearby the remains of the ancient Roman city of Volubulis where many of Morocco's agricultural traditions started,

South to the Ifrane National Park – also known as the Switzerland of Morocco, on to the Azilal province, famous for its dinosaur fossils and footprints, across the High Atlas Mountains to Ait Ben Haddou, used as a backdrop to films like Gladiator. Further south still to the desert sand dunes around Zagora, the towards the dramatic Atlantic coast and towns like Mireleft to watch the rolling waves crash against imposing cliffs.

Morocco is a country of diverse and stunning landscapes. What is consistent throughout the country, however, is the warm welcome given to travellers where the traditional greeting of 'As-salaam Alaykum' (literally – 'peace be with you'), always results in a warm smile.

This was when we discovered the rich agricultural regions stretching from the northwest to the central regions nestling in the foothills of the Atlas Mountains that have been supplying local markets with fresh produce for generations.

Morocco is a 'Garden of Eden' on the doorstep of Europe and a wonderful source of traditionally cultivated, natural, healthy produce, rich in nutrients as well as exciting new tastes.

Morocco can, however, be something of an administrative nightmare. When renovating our riad, we met Jaouad Hadani, a Moroccan-based accountant specializing in servicing English-speaking clients in Marrakech. He also has strong family connections to the Moroccan agricultural sector and prior to his accountancy career, he was responsible for organising local logistics to bring produce to market, including - his family olive oil.

Linda has always been extremely health conscious and looks after our own diet most carefully. With the growing consumer interest in and demand for pure, natural food products as part of a drive for healthy eating and living, together with care for the environment and sustainable producer methods, we saw Morocco and quality Moroccan produce as ideally placed to service these needs.

Issues Within The Olive Oil Market

Blight & Drought

From around 2014 onward, unusual weather and a proliferation of insects and bacterial blight devastated the harvest in several of the major European countries. Farmers in Italy suffered so badly from pests and adverse weather that many reported harvests down by 40% to 50%.

Adulteration & Fraud

A number of high-profile prosecutions for fraud, had also reduced consumer confidence in extra virgin olive oil products. Practices including falsely labelling poor quality oils as extra virgin; marketing olive oils from different countries / origins as (for example) 'Italian'; mixing oils of dubious provenance; using vegetable oils disguised using artificial colouring and additives (1,2).

Supermarket Behaviour

The CEO of one of the major suppliers of olive oil was recently quoted as saying – "the olive oil industry's business model is broken. (We did at the time ask – who broke it then?) Olive oil is perceived as a traffic builder by (supermarket) retailers and, of course, volume is more important than value". He went on: "even though we are dealing with a unique product, fantastic product, in my opinion, we are confusing the consumers, we are just confusing them - it's a mess." (3)

So, we thought – if the traditional EU producer countries are struggling to satisfy customers – could Morocco 'fill the gap?'.

What We Did

We carried out extensive research, value chain analysis, and detailed business modelling. We obtained olive oil samples from around the country and visited supplier sites. Our overall aim was to help establish Morocco as an alternative source of exceptionally high-quality extra virgin olive oil that had not been tainted by some of the negative behaviours of traditional EU producing countries.

We aimed to re-establish consumer trust and confidence in extra virgin olive oil as 'the original superfood' that has stood the test of time. From the outset, we also wanted to be at the forefront of 21st century retailing by making our olive oil directly available to health-conscious food-lovers worldwide through the internet, rather than through traditional bricks and mortar wholesalers and retailers.

We then teamed up with a dear old friend whom I have known for over 40 years (who though he was about to retire!).

Bob Watson has a lifetime of experience of operations in drinks industry including brewing, distilling, soft drinks, bottled water and is a recognised industry expert. This included helping to 'clean up' the bottled water industry and raise international standards following on from some major scandals. (4)

The Morocco Gold Approach

We are delighted to bring our collective years of experience within the food and drink sector to bring this centuries old 'superfood' from this amazing new source to a worldwide audience.

Our aims are to: promote Morocco as an undiscovered source of exceptionally high quality extra virgin olive oil; support healthy eating and lifestyle choices through all-natural, genuine, high quality extra virgin olive oil; set a new standard for provenance, authenticity and the guarantee of extra virgin quality; educate consumers about olive oil as an original 'superfood', rich in health enhancing polyphenols; help to transform the olive oil sector in Morocco and bring this centuries old 'superfood' to international customers.

Why This Is So Important

In a fast-changing world it is unusual to re-discover a 'wisdom of the ancients' that is as potent now as it has been for thousands of years. It has been known for centuries that high quality extra virgin olive oil is good for your health and wellbeing. It has also been lauded across many cultures.

In ancient Rome, olive oil was used for nearly everything in relation to their health. Roman medicine takes heavily from Greek doctors, who influenced European medicine for centuries.

"Let food be thy medicine and medicine be thy food"

Hippocrates : father of modern medicine

The olive tree and olive oil are mentioned seven times in the "Quran", and the olive is praised as a precious fruit. The Prophet is reported to have said: "Take olive oil and massage with it – it is a blessed tree." Early Middle Eastern civilisations relied on olive oil to cure everything. To this day, many in the region drink olive oil daily to keep the body running efficiently.

The difference now is - following extensive scientific research we now know exactly what is in high quality olive oils that are so good for you – its antioxidant polyphenols.

Morocco Gold is an exceptionally high-quality extra virgin olive oil from a unique new source. What makes it so special is it is teeming with health enhancing polyphenols. The following illustrates the range of chronic conditions where research into these polyphenols has demonstrated positive effects.

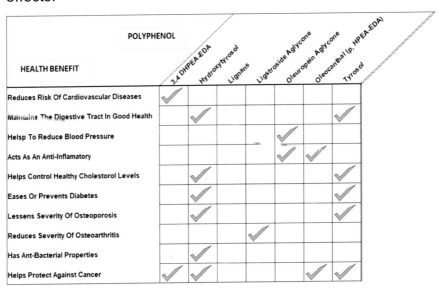

HEALTH BENEFIT	3,4 DHPEA.EDA	Hydroxytyrosol	Lignans	Ligstroside Aglycone	Oleuropein Aglycone	Oleocanthal (p, HPEA.EDA)	Tyrosol
Reduces Risk Of Cardiovascular Diseases	✓						
Maintains The Digestive Tract In Good Health		✓				✓	
Helsp To Reduce Blood Pressure				✓			
Acts As An Anti-Inflamatory				✓	✓		
Helps Control Healthy Cholestorol Levels		✓				✓	
Eases Or Prevents Diabetes		✓				✓	
Lessens Severity Of Osteoporosis		✓				✓	
Reduces Severity Of Osteoarthritis			✓				
Has Ant-Bacterial Properties		✓					
Helps Protect Against Cancer	✓	✓				✓	✓

In fact, the European Food Safety Authority has now approved health claims for extra virgin olive oils with polyphenol content of more than 250mg / kg. Morocco Gold contains polyphenols well above this level. (5)

The cost of these chronic disease to national economies is astronomic. For example, in 2016, the cost of cardiovascular diseases in the USA alone was around $555Bn. This is expected to rise to $1.1Tr by 2035. The cost to the individual, both in terms of costs of treatment, as well as the pain and suffering experienced is also huge.

Morocco Gold is on a mission to re-establish extra virgin olive oil as a healthy diet / lifestyle choice; show wellness conscious people on how this incredibly simple diet / lifestyle choice – inclusion of a high-quality extra virgin olive oil – can have a profound impact on their health and wellbeing; show how extra virgin olive fits into a wider wellness lifestyle.

We are delighted with the reception that Morocco Gold has had to date. We are equally delighted to contribute to the country we now call home. At a time when national and cross-cultural tensions are rising it is wonderful to create a cross cultural venture where people of 'good heart' can come together to create something that people from all different cultures and backgrounds can benefit from.

CHAPTER 1.
OLIVE OIL HISTORY

How It Began

Fossil evidence indicates the olive tree had its origins some 20–40 million years ago in the Oligocene era. Evidence of the first olive cultivation has been found on the border between Turkey and Syria, in the period around 6000-8000 years ago. A recent DNA study of fossilized pollen has helped to narrow it down to this period.

For thousands of years olive oil's main function was for lighting lamps rather than culinary use. Edible olives seem to date back to around the Bronze age (3150 to 1200 BCE). Over the ages the cultivation of olives and olive oil pressing managed to decrease the bitterness in olives and olive oil, also increase production.

Inventory logs carried by ancient trading ships dating back to around 4,000 BCE contain the first written records of olive oil, which was transported through the Mediterranean area from one port to another. As far back as 3000 BC, olives were grown commercially in Crete and olive oil may well have been the source of the wealth of the Minoan civilization. An olive tree near the Palace of Knossos on Crete is reputed to be around 4,000 years old.

The first great expansion of olive cultivation seems to be around Greece and Egypt around 1,700 BCE. Around 1,000 BCE the Phoenicians are thought to have brought olives to Spain and Northern Africa.

The expansion of the Roman Empire in around 900 BCE was key to the increase of olive oil and its uses. The Roman Empire expanded its civilization throughout southern Europe and North Africa, bringing with it olive trees to all conquered territories. As an important commodity, the Romans made many improvements in olive tree cultivation, olive oil extraction and storage – and valued olive oil to such an extent that it was even accepted as payment for taxes. More olive mills were built and production increased greatly as this culinary staple became more popular. The decline of the Roman Empire in 500 A.D. brought with it a decrease in olive cultivation and a reduction in olive oil use.

Olive Oil Culture: The Wisdom Of The Ancient World

Olive oil has long been considered sacred. The olive branch was often a symbol of abundance, glory, and peace. Over the years, the olive has also been used to symbolize wisdom, fertility, power, and purity.

Olive oil was used for not only food and cooking, but also lighting, sacrificial offerings, ointment, and ceremonial anointment for priestly or royal office. The leafy branches of the olive tree were ritually offered to deities and powerful figures as emblems of benediction and purification, and they were used to crown the victors of friendly games and bloody wars.

The olive tree is one of the first plants mentioned in the Christian Old Testament, and one of the most significant. An olive branch was brought back to Noah by a dove to demonstrate that the flood was over.

Ancient Greece

Olive oil was used to anoint kings and athletes in ancient Greece. It was burnt in the sacred lamps of temples and fueled the "eternal flame" of the original Olympic games. Victors in these games were crowned with its leaves.

In ancient battles, olive branches were used to crown the victors. Greek soldiers are said to have rubbed olive oil into their bodies for grooming and good health as well as using it in their lamps for lighting.

The Spartans buried their dead on a bed of olive twigs to protect their souls. The olive tree was also used to protect the living, with those who attended funerals wearing crowns of olive branches to guard themselves against evil.

Legend has it that Poseidon, the sea god, and Athena, goddess of wisdom, competed to find the gift that would be most valuable to humankind. Poseidon offered the horse and Athena the olive tree. Because of its many uses, the provision of heat, food, medicine and perfume, the olive tree was chosen as the most valuable and in return for Athena's contribution, the most powerful city in Greece was named Athens in her honour.

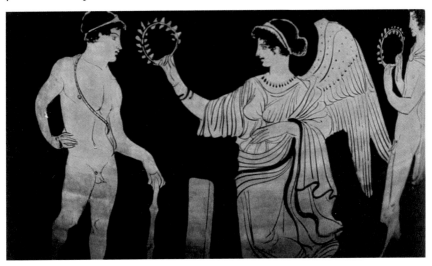

In Greece 500 B.C, olive oil's revered status was further confirmed by an image of the goddess Athena, with her head crowned with olive oil, imprinted onto the Drachma, the Greek coin. At the time, the Drachma was the Mediterranean's most circulated currency.

Ancient Rome

According to Pliny the Elder, a vine, a fig tree, and an olive tree grew in the middle of the Roman Forum; the latter was planted to provide shade.

Soaps were not around in the times of the Roman Empire. Instead, when Romans went to bathe, they rubbed olive oil all over their bodies and then scraped it off with a strigil, carrying away all the dirt and grime with it and leaving the skin silky and moisturized.

In richer patrician households, olive oil was often scented like a perfume, which would leave behind a sweet smell after it was gone. Like now, they would even pour some olive oil into their private baths to relax in them, to soften their skin and relax with some good aromatherapy.

While working out and in official competitions, athletes would rub olive oil all over their skin to make it slicker and smoother. One could also imagine how pleasing this look was to the crowd's eye in an age where physical perfection of the body was praised and immortalized in statues.

In Rome, olive oil was used for nearly everything in relation to their health. Roman medicine takes heavily from Greek doctors, who influenced European medicine for centuries, and Hippocrates, the father of modern medicine writes about over 60 different conditions or ailments that can be treated with olive oil, including skin problems, burns and wounds, ear infections, gynaecological problems, healing surgical scars, and much more. Many of these uses are still valid and are used as home remedies today.

The World's Oldest Bottle Of Olive Oil

Following a series of studies, researchers were able to confirm that the contents of a 2,000-year-old bottle found at an archaeological site in the ancient Roman town of Herculaneum, near modern-day Naples was indeed olive oil. The discovery sheds new light on the oil's molecular evolution over the past two millennia. (6)

"We are very satisfied with the insights obtained from the studies," said Raffaele Sacchi, the chair of the Food Science and Technology Unit of the University of Naples Federico II Department of Agriscience.

Working with colleagues at the National Research Council and the University of Campania Luigi Vanvitelli, Sacchi came to this conclusion after carrying out magnetic resonance and mass spectrophotometry testing on the bottle, as well as radiocarbon dating the organic residue.

"We have been able to unequivocally confirm that what we have in our hand is the most ancient olive oil residue recovered, in a significant amount, as it dates back to 79 A.D.," Sacchi said. "Moreover, our study strikingly highlights the molecular evolution of olive oil through an almost 2,000-year-long storage period."

Due to both the high temperatures caused by the eruption of Mount Vesuvius in 79 A.D. and an almost two-millennia storage period in uncontrolled conditions, the remains of the oil still bear the traces of the chemical modifications typical of altered dietary fats.

Olive Oil: A Roman Luxury Product

This amazing find also gives an insight into the value our ancient ancestors placed on olive oil. At the beginning of the first century AD, the time this bottle dates from, there was still no Latin word for glass.

Glass working was introduced to Roman culture from the Hellenistic world using their techniques and styles. Most manufacturing techniques were time-consuming, and the initial product was a thick-walled vessel which required considerable finishing. This, combined with the cost of importing natron (a naturally occurring mixture of sodium carbonate, sodium chloride and sodium sulphate) for the production of raw glass, contributed to the limited use of glass and its position as an expensive and high-status material.

So, we may conclude that the olive oil contained in this particular bottle may well have been of a very high quality and used for all the health enhancing and wellbeing benefits we enjoy from today's extra virgin olive oils like Morocco Gold.

Is Olive Oil A Food Or A Medicine?

In Rome, olive oil was used for nearly everything in relation to their health. Roman medicine takes heavily from Greek doctors, who influenced European medicine for centuries, and Hippocrates, the father of modern medicine writes about over 60 different conditions or ailments that can be treated with olive oil, including skin problems, burns and wounds, ear infections, gynaecological problems, healing surgical scars, and much more. Many of these uses are still valid and are used as home remedies today.

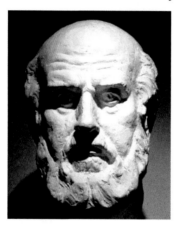

"Let food be thy medicine and medicine be thy food"

Hippocrates: father of modern medicine

The Roman doctor Galen, who was born in Greece, was also credited with the invention of cold cream, using olive oil as his base instead of the modern-day mineral oil. It has been in used for over a thousand years for soothing skin and relieving sunburns.

Olive Oil & Islam

The olive tree and olive oil are mentioned seven times in the Quran, and the olive is praised as a precious fruit. Olive trees and olive-oil health benefits have been propounded in Prophetic medicine. The Prophet is reported to have said: "Take olive oil and massage with it – it is a blessed tree."

Early Middle Eastern civilisations relied on Olive Oil to cure everything. To this day, many in the region drink olive oil daily to keep the body running efficiently. Warm olive oil is commonly used in the west to soothe earaches.

Olive oil was believed to bestow strength and youth, not least because of the tree's longevity and its tremendous resilience. Even through the harshest summers and winters, they continue to grow strong and bear fruit

A Celtic Connection

Archaeologists studying early Celtic remain in France (7) have discovered traces of olive oil on pottery fragments dating from around 500 BCE, providing the earliest known evidence of olive oil use in Central Europe. Previously, the earliest evidence for olive oil use was from the Roman period, several centuries later.

The discovery was made while examining the remains of 99 ceramic vessels from the hill fortress of Mont Lassois in Burgundy, east-central France. Traces of organic substances were found on the vessels, including beeswax, beer, wine, millet, milk, and olive oil.

The study was conducted by an international team of researchers, led by archaeologist Philipp Stockhammer from the Ludwig-Maximillian's-Universität München.

"As the sixth century BCE is the first time that Mediterranean pottery was brought to Central Europe in large amounts, I think that it is most probable that we found the earliest evidence"- *Philipp Stockhammer, an archaeologist from Ludwig-Maximillian's-Universität München.*

The early Celts inhabited southern Germany, northern Switzerland, and part of eastern France during the Early Iron Age. It has long been known that they traded with Mediterranean communities, adopting not only their goods but also some of their traditions, such as wine-feasting. What was not known until now was that olive oil was among the foreign imports.

While the researchers are confident that the oil was imported from the Mediterranean coast of France, they still do not know where it was produced.

According to the study, which was published in the scientific journal Plos in June 2020, the Celts travelled south along the Rhone River to trade with Greek colonies on the French coast, particularly Marseille, bringing back a range of Mediterranean goods. These imports included Greek and Italian pottery, as well as grape wine, and olive oil.

"The imports came via Marseille," Stockhammer said. "But we have imported vessels from the southern Greek mainland, southern Italy, and southern France, all of them possible origins of the olive oil, too."

Of the 99 vessels examined, 16 were imports, while 83 were made locally by the Celts. According to Maxime Rageot from the University of Tübingen, who conducted the food residue analysis, olive oil was found on both the imports and locally made vessels, suggesting the Celts actually used the olive oil.

Rageot used gas chromatography and GC-mass spectrometry analyses in his work. While such technology can identify organic substances with some accuracy, the job is often more difficult with older samples. "The issue of degradation, which particularly affects the lipids found in plant oils, means it is difficult to determine how widespread olive oil use was" he said.

"We have only rarely found evidence of olive oil in archaeological contexts based on organic residues, because the specific molecular markers of most plant oils are not very stable over time, and only in good contexts for lipid preservation," he added.

"So, it is not yet possible to say if olive oil was commonly imported into central Europe during the Early Iron Age or if it was a rare and very prestigious good restricted to the Celtic elites," he added.

He said this also poses problems in identifying how the olive oil was used. While most modern consumers view olive oil as a foodstuff, ancient cultures often found other uses for it.

Stock hammer said that the findings do not indicate how the oil was used, but it was likely for "body embalmment; most probably not for cooking."

The study is an important addition to the history of olive oil, showing how and when it spread north from the Mediterranean. Relatively speaking, the Celts were late in adopting the substance.

Olive Oil Rediscovered

Around 1,110 AD, olive groves began to flourish once again, particularly in Italy, thanks to the merchant class who discovered that selling olive oil in local markets was an important source of income. During this time, Tuscany becomes a renowned region for the cultivation of olive trees. During the Renaissance, Italy becomes the largest producer of olive oil in the world, renowned for its rich and flavourful oils that graced the tables of nobles and royalty throughout Europe.

Olive Oil And The New World

Spanish colonists brought the olive to the New World in the 16th century where its cultivation prospered in present-day Peru and Chile. Olive tree cultivation quickly spread along the valleys of South America's dry Pacific coast where the climate was similar to the Mediterranean. Spanish missionaries established olive trees in the 18th century in California. It was first cultivated at Mission San Diego de Alcalá in 1769 or later around 1795.

Around 1,800 AD, olive oil made its commercial debut in the Americas as Italian and Greek immigrants demanded its import from Europe.

Currently, olive oil continues to grow in popularity as an important ingredient in everyday cuisines. Consumption is still predominantly in Mediterranean countries with a long tradition of olive oil culture however as more countries are becoming health conscious, olive oil is re-asserting itself as the original super-food, thanks to its proven health benefits and nutritional properties.

Are All Olive Oils The Same?

Olives are fruit grown on the olive tree, olea europaea. There are six natural subspecies of *Olea europaea* that are now distributed over increasingly wide geographical regions.

Olea europaea (Mediterranean Basin)

Olea europaea var. *sylvestris*, considered the "wild" olive of the Mediterranean, is a variety characterized by a smaller tree bearing noticeably smaller fruit.

Olea europaea cuspidate (South Africa, throughout East Africa, Arabia to South-West China)

Olea europaea subsp. *guanchica* (Canaries)

Olea europaea subsp. *cerasiformis* (Madeira)

Olea europaea subsp. *maroccana* (Morocco)

Olea europaea subsp. *laperrinei* (Algeria, Sudan, Niger)

Wild growing forms of the olive are sometimes treated as the species Olea oleaster. In recent times, efforts have been directed at producing hybrid cultivars with qualities useful to farmers, such as resistance to disease, quick growth, and larger or more consistent crops.

There are now hundreds of cultivars of the olive tree are known. An olive cultivar has a significant impact on its colour, size, shape, and growth characteristics, as well as the qualities of olive oil. Olive cultivars may be used primarily for olive oil, eating, or both.

As a result of its ongoing success, there are now more than 860 million olive trees in the world today, with more being planted every day! Each cultivar is enhanced and improved for flavour, stability, and size. There are over 700 varieties across the world today.

I ike wines, extra virgin olive oils can vary dramatically in taste, depending upon the type and quality of the fruit that is pressed, the time of harvest, the weather during the growing season, and the region from which the olives were produced.

Connoisseurs generally use the following in appraising extra virgin olive oils: mild, semi-fruity, and fruity, depending on the flavour of the olive that can be detected.

Types Of Olive Oil

There are five different types of olive oil:

1. Extra Virgin Olive Oil

2. Virgin Olive Oil

3. Refined Olive Oil

4. Olive Pomace Oil

5. Lampante Oil

Extra Virgin Olive Oil: The Highest Quality Olive Oil

Extra virgin olive oil is a wholly natural, unrefined oil and the highest quality olive oil you can buy. Genuine extra virgin olive oil is rare and as a result is slightly more expensive.

Because of the way extra virgin olive oil is made, it retains a truer olive taste and has a lower level of oleic acid (no more than 0.8%) than other olive oil varieties. It also contains more of the natural vitamins and minerals found in olives.

Extra virgin olive oil is completely natural. It is not treated with chemicals or altered by temperature. It typically has a golden-green colour, with a distinctive fresh, green flavour and a light peppery finish.

How the fruit was grown, harvested, and transported, how it was pressed into oil, and how the oil was packaged and bottled all contribute to ensuring extra virgin olive oil like Morocco Gold is the best quality olive oil you can buy.

The definition of extra virgin olive oil is very precise regards production methods, taste, and chemical composition. To be certified as extra virgin, an olive oil must:

Come from a single source, it is not mixed/blended with other olive oils, even if they are of extra virgin quality

Come from the first pressing of fresh, young olives, normally within 24 hours of harvesting

Be extracted purely by mechanical means at temperatures specifically below 28C.

Have free fatty acid or acidity level (normally measured as oleic acid) of less than 0.8%.

Be defect free and have a perfect taste and aroma.

Extra virgin olive oil is also the healthiest, providing a wide range of health benefits. High-quality extra virgin olive oils like Morocco Gold contain antioxidants, in particular polyphenols that provide the health-enhancing qualities associated with olive oil.

Virgin Olive Oil

Next in quality is virgin olive oil. It is made using a similar process as extra virgin olive oil and is also an unrefined oil, meaning chemicals or heat are not used to extract oil from the fruit. Virgin olive oil also maintains the purity and taste of the olive, though production standards are not as rigid.

According to the standards of the International Olive Council, virgin olive oil has a slightly higher level of oleic acid of up to 2%. It also has a slightly less intense flavour than extra-virgin olive oil. Virgin oil is rarely found, if ever, however, in grocery stores; usually, your choice will be between extra virgin, regular, and light olive oils.

Refined Olive Oil

These are olive oils that have been refined by using agents such as acids, alkalis, and heat to extract as much oil as possible from the olive pulp that remains after the first pressing. The result is a fattier and more acidic oil which lacks taste, aroma, and natural antioxidants found in extra virgin olive oil.

Producers then need to add unrefined extra virgin or virgin olive oil to give refined olive oil some flavour, colour, and aroma into the blend. Terms such as "pure" or "100% pure" or "Light" are made-up terms used by large producers and supermarkets. If the label states "pure" or "100% pure" or "Light" then the olive oil is a refined oil lacking the taste, aroma and quality of extra virgin olive oil.

Olive Pomace Oil

The lowest grade of olive oil made from the by-products of extra virgin olive oil production. Olive skins, seeds, and pulp are heated, and the remaining oil is extracted using solvent. The result, pomace oil, is then put through a refining process, similar to pure or light olive oil.

Pomace olive oil is bland and extremely low in antioxidants.

Lampante Oil

Lampante oil comes from bad fruit or poor processing practices and has severe taste defects. It is not fit for human consumption until it has been refined.

Extra Virgin Olive Oil: What Factors Determine The Taste

High quality extra virgin olive oil is like fine wine, there is an incredibly wide choice and taste. Each olive oil has its own unique taste characteristics depending on the type of olive or varietal the olive oil comes from, the soil conditions where the olive trees are grown, when the olives are harvested, how the olives are treated during the harvesting and pressing to produce the olive oil and a whole host of other factors.

For example, oil made from predominantly unripe (green) olives contain flavours described as grassy, artichoke, or tomato leaf, whereas riper olives tend to yield softer flavours often described as buttery floral or tropical.

The above descriptions are associated with high-quality, extra virgin olive, but trained tasters also learn to identify negative characteristics. Flavour defects in olive oil are associated with problems with the olive fruit (olive fly, frozen conditions), improper handling of olives during harvest (dirt, wet fruit, prolonged storage prior to milling), certain milling conditions (unsanitary equipment, excessive heat), and improper or prolonged storage after milling (oxidation).

Olive oil that is determined to have flavour defects is not of genuine extra virgin quality. According to the International Olive Council extra virgin olive oil must meet both chemical and organoleptic (flavour) standards that include the absence of flavour defects.

The first step in learning how to taste olive oil is to understand how our senses work. Perception of flavour relies on both our senses of taste and smell. The ability to taste is quite limited; receptors on our tongue can only discern sweet, salt, sour, bitter, and umami (the flavour of protein). All other information that we think of as flavour is actually perceived by smelling food through the back of our nostrils (retro-nasally) while it is in our mouths. To illustrate this fact, think about how little flavour we perceive when we have a cold (or indeed now Covid!). This is because one cannot smell food retro-nasally when one's nose is stuffed up.

Tasting Olive Oil

When tasting extra virgin olive oil, much of the olive oil's characteristics are perceived through the sense of smell. Though most people enjoy olive oil with other foods, the following steps allow us to focus on the olive oil's flavour without distraction:

Pour a small amount of olive oil (about 1 tablespoon) into a small tapered (wine) glass.

Hold the glass in one hand and use your other hand to cover the glass while swirling the olive oil to release its aroma.

Uncover the glass and inhale deeply from the top of the glass. Think about whether the aroma is mild or strong. You may want to write down descriptions of the aromas that you detect at this point.

Next, you slurp the olive oil. This is done by sipping a small amount of olive oil into your mouth while "sipping" some air as well. (When done correctly, you will make that impolite noise that would cause you to be scolded when you were a child!) Slurping emulsifies the olive oil with air that helps to spread it throughout your mouth, giving you the chance to savour every nuance of flavour with just a small sip of oil.

Finish by swallowing the olive oil and noticing if it leaves a stinging sensation in your throat.

Each of the above actions focuses our attention on a specific positive attribute in the olive oil. Firstly, we evaluate the olive fruit aroma (fruitiness) by inhaling from the glass. When the olive oil is in our mouth, we further evaluate the aroma retro-nasally as well as determine the amount of bitterness on our tongues. Lastly, we determine the intensity of the olive oil's pungency in our throats as we swallow it.

Does The Colour Of The Olive Oil Matter?

The olive oil colour is not addressed during a sensory assessment. The reason is that contrary to the common belief that golden olive oil is mild and dark green olive oil is robust, colour is NOT an indicator of either the olive oil's flavour or quality. In fact, in scientific assessments, we sample from specially designed blue glasses that obscure the colour of the olive oil. Tasting from a dark glass prevents us from having preconceptions about the flavour of the olive oil before we can actually smell or taste it.

Practice Tasting Olive Oil

Once you are comfortable with the above tasting method, try the following exercise. Select three olive oils labelled as extra virgin olive oil, including an inexpensive imported brand from the supermarket. In between samples, clean your palate by eating a small piece of tart, green apple and then rinsing your mouth with water.

Consider the following as you evaluate each olive oil sample:

Is the aroma of the olive oil pleasant or unpleasant?

Is the olive oil aroma mild, strong, or somewhere in the middle (we'll call that medium)? When assessing the second and third olive oils, note if the aroma's intensity is weaker or stronger than the previous sample.

Note 3 words (or phrases) that describe the aroma.

Is the olive oil bitter, which is primarily sensed towards the back of the tongue? Would you describe the bitterness of the olive oil as mild, medium, or strong? Is the intensity of the olive oil's bitterness in balance with the intensity of the aroma?

When you swallow the olive oil, how does it feel in your throat? Did the oil leave a mild impression, or did it sting your throat or make you cough? Is the intensity of the oil's pungency in balance with the olive oil's aroma and bitterness?

When you have completed the above exercise, take a few moments to review your notes. What were the characteristics that you enjoyed the most? Were there any characteristics of the olive oil that you didn't enjoy? How did the supermarket brand compare to the other olive oils? Even without an experienced taster sharing their thoughts about the olive oils with you, there is much you can learn by tasting olive oils on your own.

Using this same tasting method, you can sample another set of oils on another day and still be able to compare your responses to the first set; this is how we build our personal olive oil "vocabulary". You will begin to recognize flavours and may even discover which varietals produce the flavours you prefer.

You will learn to compare the level of intensity for fruity aroma, bitterness, and pungency and will begin to identify olive oils as mild, medium, and robust (intense). It's a good idea to organize your tasting notes in a binder so you can review your past tasting experiences with new ones.

Taste is personal, so not everyone will agree on which varietals, and other factors, produce the best olive oil. However, tasting oils in a methodical fashion will help to educate your palate, and you will be able to select oils with flavour characteristics that you enjoy and enhance your meals.

Here is a list of terms commonly used to define olive oil taste, positive and negative. (8)

Positive Attributes: Extra Virgin Olive Oil

Apple/Green Apple: Indicative of certain olive varietals

Almond: Nutty (fresh not oxidized)

Artichoke: Green flavour

Astringent: Puckering sensation in mouth created by tannins; often associated with bitter, robust oils

Banana: Ripe and unripe banana fruit

Bitter: Considered a positive attribute because it is indicative of fresh olive fruit

Buttery: Creamy, smooth sensation on palate

Eucalyptus: Aroma of specific olive varietals

Floral: Perfume/aroma of flowers

Forest: Fresh aroma reminiscent of forest floor, NOT dirty

Fresh: Good aroma, fruity, not oxidized

Fruity: Refers to the aroma of fresh olive fruit, which is perceived through the nostrils and retro-nasally when the oil is in one's mouth.

Grass: The aroma of fresh-cut (mowed) grass

Green/Greenly: Aroma/flavour of unripe olives

Green Tea: Characteristic of some unripe olive varieties

Harmonious: Balance among the oil's characteristics with none overpowering the others

Hay/Straw: Dried grass flavour

Herbaceous: Unripe olive fruit reminiscent of fresh green herbs

Melon: Indicative of certain olive varietals

Mint: Indicative of certain olive varietals

Pear: Indicative of certain olive varietals

Peach: Indicative of certain olive varietals

Peppery: Stinging sensation in the throat which can force a cough (see pungent)

Pungent: Stinging sensation in the throat which can force a cough (see peppery)

Ripely: Aroma/flavour of ripe olive fruit

Round/Rotund: A balanced, mouth-filling sensation of harmonious flavours

Spice: Aroma/flavour of seasonings such as cinnamon, allspice (but not herbs or pepper)

Sweet: Characteristic of mild oils

Tomato Leaf: Indicative of certain olive varietals

Tropical: Indicative of ripe olive fruit with nuances of melon, mango, and coconut

Walnut Shell: Nutty (fresh not oxidized)

Wheatgrass: Strong flavour of some green olive fruit

Woody: Indicative of olive varietals with large pits

Negative Attributes: Non-Extra Virgin Olive Oil

Acetone: Aroma of nail polish remover, associated with winey defect

Blue Cheese: Aroma associated with muddy sediment defect

Brine: Salty taste indicating that oil was made from brined olives

Bacon: Smoky essence that may indicate oxidation

Burnt/Heated: Caused by processing at too high a temperature

Cucumber: Off flavour from prolonged storage, particularly in tin

Dirty: Oils which have absorbed unpleasant odours and flavours of dirty wastewater during milling

Dreggish: Odour of warm lubricating oil caused by the poor execution of the decanting process

Esparto: Refers to straw-like material in mats occasionally used in older mills that may create a hemp-like flavour in oil

Fiscolo: Refers to coconut fibres in mats occasionally used in older mills that may create a hemp-like flavour in oil

Flat/Bland: Oils which have no positive or negative aroma or flavour characteristic of olive oil; may indicate presence of refined olive oil

Frozen/Wet Wood: Sweet, dry, and untypical aroma/flavour derived from olives which have been exposed to freezing temperatures

Fusty: Anaerobic fermentation that occurs when olives are stored in piles too long before milling

Greasy: Flavour of diesel or gasoline caused by equipment problems

Grubby: Flavour imparted to oil by olive fly damage to olives

Hay-wood: Flavour of dried olives

Muddy Sediment: Barnyard-like aroma caused by olives' prolonged contact with dirt before or after milling

Musty: Mouldy, humid flavour created by wet olives that have been stored too long before pressing

Metallic: Oils that have had prolonged contact with reactive metal surfaces either during processing or storage

Rancid: The flavour of oxidation that occurs as the oil ages, often described as "stale nuts"

Rough: Pasty, thick, greasy mouth feel

Sour Milk: Aroma associated with muddy sediment defect

Stale Nuts: Flavour of oxidized oils, rancidity

Unbalanced: Oils with overwhelming flavours of bitterness and pungency

Vegetable Water: Oils that have been stored in contact with the water content of the olive after processing

Winey: Sour/vinegary flavour caused by aerobic fermentation of olives during processing (see vinegary)

Vinegary: Sour/vinegary flavour caused by aerobic fermentation of olives during processing. (see winey)

Yeasty: Aroma of bread dough; associated with winey defect

CHAPTER 2.
MOROCCO: A RICH HERITAGE OF OLIVE OIL PRODUCTION

Morocco has been producing high quality olive oil for millennia, from the time of the Romans. The existence of centenary trees and traditional presses (maasras), testify to the antiquity of olive oil production. Indeed, olive oil has long been considered a noble food by the local population.

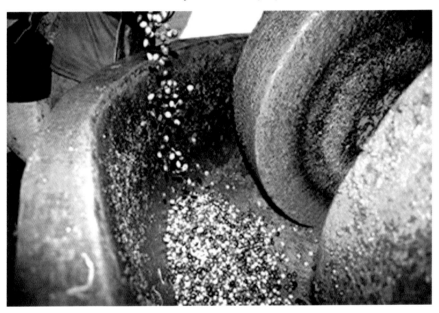

The benign climate makes Morocco a 'Garden Of Eden' on the doorstep of Europe and the ideal location for olive cultivation with mild winters and warm, dry summers. The soils in the main olive-growing regions are rich and deep and generally have an equal balance of clay and coarse sands.

However, despite now being the fourth largest producer of olives in the world (Morocco harvested an estimated 2 million tons of olives in the 2018/19 harvest), the quality of Moroccan olive oil has until now been relatively little known outside of the country.

Researchers, using International Olive Council standards, published a report on the quality and purity of Moroccan olive oil in the journal Food Chemistry. They classified 94 percent of samples tested as extra virgin olive oil and only 6 percent as virgin olive oil.

Morocco Gold extra virgin olive oil comes from groves in the foothills of the Atlas Mountains. The specific soil conditions of the Beni Mellal region, together with the mild winters and summers caressed by hot winds from the Sahara, make ideal growing conditions for Morocco Gold olives.

Nurtured with love for generations, using only traditional, natural methods, Morocco Gold retains its distinctive flavour to offer the finest sensory experience.

The Traditional Way Of Producing Olive Oil

The traditional method of extracting olive oil from the fruit is virtually the same today as it has been for thousands of years. At harvest time, which varies from region to region, olives are harvested by hand and collected in nets placed around the foot of the tree. A day or two thereafter, the olives are taken to the mill. Giant stones weighing several tons were used to crush the olives and pits into a mash.

The olive mash was then spread onto thin mats. These mats were stacked and placed into a "press." As the press applied several hundred pounds of pressure, oil and water from the mash seeped out of the mats and dripped into collection vats. In the traditional method, no heat is applied in the pressing - hence the term "first cold pressed."

Project Green

Even though olive cultivation has been part of Morocco's agricultural scene since the Roman era, and Morocco is the world's sixth-largest producer of olive oil, the quality and compositional peculiarities of Moroccan olive oil have been relatively unknown.

Morocco is already the second-largest global exporter of table olives. It is now reaping the rewards of the government's Project Green plan for olive farming. In 2008, The Moroccan Government introduced the program to encourage farmers in rural areas to switch to growing olive trees instead of wheat or other crops, creating more jobs and a boost to olive oil production. Thanks to the initiative, Morocco now has one million hectares dedicated to olive groves.

According to the Moroccan centre for Export Promotion, Morocco almost doubled its production in six years to 1.5 million tons. The olive oil sector has greatly reduced unemployment for women in particular, creating over 300,000 permanent jobs.

Over 1,000 professionals from across the country participated in a training program organized by the Moroccan Inter professional Olive Federation, in partnership with the National Office of the Agricultural Council and the National Office for the Sanitary Protection of Food Products – ONSSA. Covering topics such as productivity, quality, pests and diseases, and legal aspects, the training program was conducted on 43 sites in the olive producing regions of de Fès-Meknès, Marrakech-Safi, Béni Mellal-Khénifra, 'Oriental, Tanger-Tétouan-Al Hoceima, and Rabat-Salé-Kénitra. The ultimate objective of the program was to foster a quality production of olive products like oil and table olives.

What Makes Morocco Gold So Special

The story of Morocco Gold Extra Virgin olive oil arguably begins a long time ago – a very long time ago.

The Morocco Gold olive growing area is 280 kms and about 4-hour drive northeast of Marrakesh. It is situated in a raised valley in the foothills of the magnificent Atlas Mountains in the Azilal Province which is part of the Beni Mellal region. The area rarely sees many tourists or outsiders.

The geological history of this remote and unspoiled valley shows that it was formed in the early Jurassic period, around 190 million years ago. It shows well preserved sediments and rocks of marine origin (called Lias) towards the valley sides and sediments alternating between shallow marine carbonates, continental silts, and red sandstone from the Cretaceous era – around 145 – 66 million years ago towards the center of the valley.

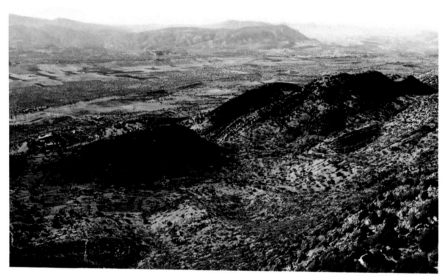

The Cretaceous covers a period with a relatively warm climate, with sea-level changes (known as tectono-eustatic oscillations) driven either by increases in the volumes of the oceans, or by the rising and falling of the land due to tectonic plate movements – a process that helped form the Atlas Mountains themselves. The evidence strongly suggests that this valley was at one time underwater.

During the Cretaceous, new groups of mammals, birds as well as flowering plants appeared. The end of the Cretaceous is also defined by the abrupt mass extinction in which many dinosaurs and large marine reptiles died out. (Interestingly, another feature of the Azilal province is the preponderance of dinosaur fossils from this period).

Over time, however, the layer upon layer of decomposed organic matter has contributed massively to the rich content of phenols in the local soil. This in turn contributes to the very high levels polyphenols found in olives now grown in the region.

This raised valley is between two 1400m Atlas ranges with altitude varying between 700m and 900m along its 40kms. This creates its own micro-climate with temperatures generally 2c below the coastal plain in the daytime and 5c at night-time. These differences, combined with the naturally occurring nutrients in the soil, create uniquely high-quality olive growing conditions for the Picholine Marocaine, the only type of olive used in Morocco Gold.

The Picholine Marocaine

The Picholine Marocaine is the only variety of olive used in the production of Morocco Gold. This olive has smooth skin, a fleshy mesocarp rich in fat, containing a woody nucleus, which contains a seed. Its color, at first green, turns black at full maturity. Maturity is reached between November and December.

Oil from the Picholine Marocaine is also recognized for its longevity and high levels of polyphenols. This makes it particularly attractive to health-conscious food lovers – worldwide. Oil from the Picholine is typically described as:

Golden yellow in colour

A fruity taste with an average intensity of more than 6 on the International Olive Council (IOC) organoleptic scale.

A taste of sweet almond, carob, fresh turf, and hint of herbs.

Degree of 'pepperiness' varies between 3 and 6 on the organoleptic scale of the IOC

The Importance Of Polyphenols

Extra virgin olive oil is probably the most extensively researched foodstuff on the planet, and the health benefits are evidence based. Thanks to the recent spotlight on the Mediterranean Diet, extensive research has been done on the phytonutrient composition of olive oil. What has been discovered is an extensive list of phytonutrients; one of the most praised is its polyphenols. The number of polyphenols found in extra virgin olive oil is truly amazing!

Polyphenols are a potent antioxidant, one that can decommission a nasty molecule in your body called free radicals. Free radicals can ricochet around inside your body and harm good cells. Antioxidants, such as the polyphenols found in extra virgin olive oil work to neutralize free radicals and so protecting the body from their harmful effects.

The high polyphenol content of Morocco Gold extra virgin olive oil is dependent on three factors. First is the variety of the olive, secondly the climate and terroir of the growing region, and thirdly the actual time in the growing season that the crop is harvested.

Morocco Gold is pressed from the Picholine Marocaine, the only type of olive to go into Morocco Gold. Oil from this variety is renowned for its high polyphenol count, oxidative stability, and longevity.

Our olives are grown in a valley that is about 2,000 feet above sea level. This helps to create the additional climatic challenges that encourage polyphenol uptake within the olive tree. It is also an area with naturally occurring high phenols in the soil itself.

In soils, phenols are released over an extended period of time from decomposing plant materials. This causes complex organic compounds to be slowly oxidized or to break down into simpler forms of sugars, amino sugars, aliphatic and phenolic organic acids. These are further transformed into microbial biomass or are reorganized, and further oxidized into humic assemblages (fulvic and humic acids), which bind to clay minerals.

There has been a long debate about the ability of plants to uptake humic substances through their root systems and to metabolize them. There is now a consensus about how humus plays a hormonal role rather than simply a nutritional role in plant physiology. Olive trees grown in 'challenging' conditions encourage the uptake of naturally occurring phenols in the soil. This, in turn aids the circulatory system within the olive tree, with the phenols eventually finding their way to the olive fruit itself.

Thirdly, our olives are picked when the fruit is young and green. As the olives age on the tree, the colour of the olive changes to red and then black, the size of the olive increases thus producing more oil, but the polyphenol level decreases. There is a great deal of expertise within the farming community where we source our oil to ensure that the harvest is collected at the optimum time to maximise the polyphenol level.

How Our Olives Are Grown

Olive trees can produce olives for hundreds of years. Yet olive trees typically alternate between bearing small crops and normal crops every other year. They can also go for 2 - 3 years without bearing any fruit. There are a number of key stages in the life cycle of the olive tree leading up to the harvesting and pressing of our extra virgin olive oil.

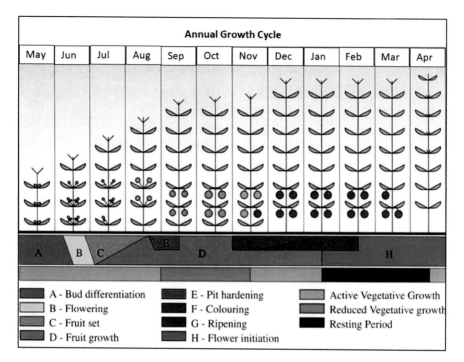

Annual Growth Cycle											
May	Jun	Jul	Aug	Sep	Oct	Nov	Dec	Jan	Feb	Mar	Apr

A - Bud differentiation
B - Flowering
C - Fruit set
D - Fruit growth

E - Pit hardening
F - Colouring
G - Ripening
H - Flower initiation

Active Vegetative Growth
Reduced Vegetative growth
Resting Period

Flowering

Olive trees produce fruiting shoots called *inflorescences* which originate at the axil of a leaf. Each inflorescence will typically contain 10 to 30 flowers, depending on the type of olive. The number of flowers that then mature into olives dependent on a number of factors.

The 'Goldilocks' Zone

Olive trees require temperatures that are – not too hot – not too cold – but just right!. They require winter cold to achieve normal blooming and fruiting. The optimal degree of cold winters is dependent upon the origin of the olive cultivar (e.g., Eastern Mediterranean vs. Southern Europe). Strong winds, hot temperatures, and freezing temperatures can negatively impact the fruit set. Particularly cold springs will negatively impact harvest by delaying blooming and increasing flower abnormalities. Localized winter temperature rises due to development around the tree, such as buildings, and asphalt can act as a wintertime heat sink, thereby inhibiting fruiting. The remote, elevated valley in the foothills of the Atlas Mountains provides the ideal balance of temperature throughout the olive growing season.

Blooming

Before flowers bloom, they go through a differentiation period that has to do with the sexuality of the blooms. This generally takes place March through May and results in one of two results (although there is some new research indicating that there may be a third possible result).

Perfect Flowers

This is where flowers have both stamen (the male part) and pistil (the female part)

Staminate Flowers

This is where flowers have only stamens and lack a pistil (which apparently have been aborted).

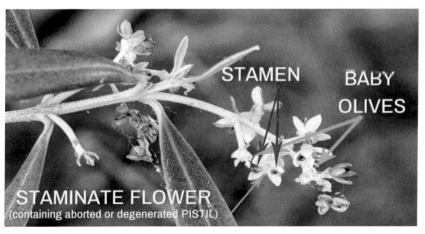

Why are there staminate flowers and not just perfect (hermaphroditic) flowers? There are a number of theories and reasons, but the main ones are thought to be:

It takes a great deal of energy to develop the pistil (or ovule - think of this as the human ovum). The tree has to moderate the number of pistils it is able to develop with the nutrients available to it.

In order to pollinate the pistil, the tree is dependent on a high volume of stamens – stamens don't have the same nutrient requirements as the pistils, so the tree exercises her "nutrient economizing" by terminating pistils (ovules) as needed.

Orchard stress, in particular water stress, can negatively impact this portion of the development. In competitions between flowers and leaves, the leaves win, and the first floral part to fail is the pistil. A moist soil profile during this period can help prevent this kind of stress.

Pistil abortion occurs naturally and is not perfectly understood. Pistil formation must compete with vegetative growth for nutrients at a time when both are working their hardest. In addition, following a big harvest year, the tree's nutritional resources have been depleted. Yet, if only 1% - 2% of the flowers are able to set fruit, the grower will still enjoy a satisfactory crop. If a tree is blooming, but no olives develop, this could be because of a mechanical disruption to the fruit set. Wind, rain, and/or hail can knock off the blooms just at this critical time of the year.

Pollination

According to the Olive Production Manual (University of California, Agriculture, and Natural Resources), "...some 500,000 flowers are present in a mature tree..." at time of full bloom. Within two weeks of full bloom, most of the flowers will have failed, with only 1 – 2% then maturing into full-grown fruit.

Self-Pollination

Because of their geometry, olive flowers self-pollinate. The anthers (located at the top of the filaments attached to the stamen) drop pollen on the stigma of the pistil. The pollen grains germinate, and olive growth is underway. Though not necessary for pollination, wind and bees may aid in pollination by disturbing the flower causing pollen to fall from the anther to the stigma. Many olive varieties cannot self-pollinate. For these trees, olive pollen is primarily carried by the wind. Bees may play a minor role in pollination.

Cross Pollination

Cross-pollination occurs when wind or a bee transfers pollen from one flower to the stigma of another flower. As bees are not particularly fond of olive flowers, they do not typically play a large role in the olive orchard.

Stress – It's Not Good For Olives Either!

As with us humans, stress on the olive tree and its fruit will be detrimental. This may be caused by a number of factors including too much or too little pruning, shortage of water – when the tree will favour the leaf over the fruit and pest infections. (9)

How It Is Done: Achieving The Best Quality Oil

Our aim was to bring the highest quality extra virgin olive oil from this amazing, undiscovered source to health concious food lovers worldwide through ethically sourced, environmentally sustainable means.

The specific soil conditions of the Beni Mellal region, together with the mild winters and summers caressed by hot winds from the Sahara, make ideal growing conditions for Morocco Gold olives. The existence of centenary trees and traditional presses (maasras) testify to the longevity of olive cultivation in this area.

Olives from the Beni-Mellal region have been grown for centuries using traditional farming methods. The exceptionally high quality of Morocco Gold extra virgin olive oil is the result of care and attention to detail throughout the entire production process.

Groundwork and tillage are carried out once or twice a year: once in winter to facilitate rainwater infiltration into the soil, and in spring to rotate the soil.

Planting is done at the beginning of spring. There is some permitted intercropping of cereals, also almond trees, that contribute to the hint of almonds in Morocco Gold.

In addition to natural rainfall, which is generally sufficient in the geographical area, trees are irrigated as needed during the period of vegetation of the olive tree, normally until the end of September.

Fruiting sizing and assessment of the maturity of the olive are carried out annually. The planned date of harvest is agreed based on the maturity index of the olives also the generations of experience of the olive farmers. Harvesting will then normally take place between the end of October and beginning of December.

Harvesting Morocco Gold Olives

If you're a farmer, the word *harvest* elicits myriad emotions. Feelings range from stress to anxiety to relief and to hope and joy. And if you are fortunate enough to allow yourself a few spare moments during this exhausting season, you might just find yourself overwhelmed with a feeling of contentment and satisfaction rarely found in our modern world.

Determining when to harvest is not an exact science. It is an amalgam of a number of factors such as the desired olive oil yield, intended level of antioxidants, and, of course, the desired flavour profile.

It is important to strike the right balance for Morocco Gold customers. Our aim is to combine the taste characteristics of a premium extra virgin olive oil, young and fruity, with the health enhancing polyphenols to create an extra virgin olive oil that is well balanced and not too 'aggressive' when taken on its own.

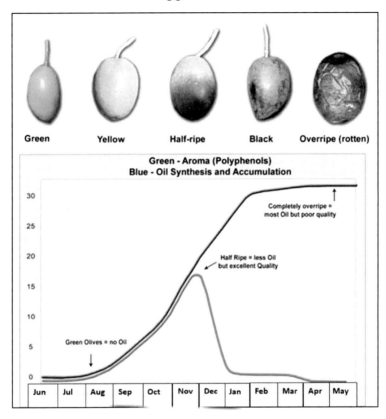

Green — Aroma (Polyphenols)
Blue — Oil Synthesis and Accumulation

A key to achieving this balance is the generations of experience of our olive growers, the care and attention they pay to their crop throughout the whole growing season, and the dedication and attention to detail paid during the harvesting process. We have been extremely fortunate to work with local experts to determine the exact right time to harvest

Harvesting requires a lot of preparation and planning including having our dedicated team of women harvesters, the 'sisterhood' ready and eager, the harvesting equipment in working order, transportation arranged to carry our olives to the mill, are just a few of the preparations that need to be in place.

Morocco Gold olives are harvested by hand using flexible combs. Nets and tarpaulins are placed on the ground to avoid contact between the olives and the ground.

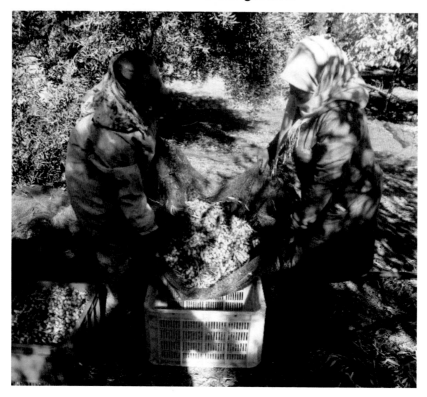

When you see those first mounds of olives accumulating in the harvest trays, it's a magical moment. It's like you've been transformed into the richest person in all the land. Yet we all know that none of us are in this business for the money – it's about the richness of the journey. The thing that I have been working for all year is finally coming to fruition. Incidentally, the word itself derives from the Latin fruit ("to use, enjoy") and fruit (sense of "act or state of bearing fruit"). When the fruit is finally being plucked off the trees and collected into trays for milling, it is truly a joyous occasion. There's a sense of excitement around your hopes for a solid yield with superior flavour.

Aerated boxes are used for the immediate transport of the harvested olives from the orchard to the crushing unit. On receipt, the olives are checked to ensure their quality, in particular color and appearance, any defective or malformed olives.

The olives will then pass through a stripper to remove any impurities. They are then washed and drained before processing. Leaf stripping and washing eliminate impurities, whether of vegetable origins such as leaves, twigs, or mineral matter such as dust, earth, stones, and other solids. Washing improves not only the quality of the product but also extraction efficiency.

Extraction of oil is carried out in a continuous two-phase process. This minimizes handling of the olives and maintains strict control of hygiene.

Grinding of the olives is carried out using a metal hammer mill which is made of stainless steel. The paste obtained then undergoes a kneading or malaxation process which is the fundamental operation to separate the solid and liquid phases. This kneading operation is carried out for 40 to 50 minutes at temperatures not exceeding 28 ° C. In this way, the extracted oil may be labeled: cold-extracted oil or cold-pressed oil.

The well-kneaded dough is sent to a horizontal decanter where the continuous and simultaneous separation of the oil and wet cakes is achieved by a combination of centrifugal force and of the rotation of a conveyor screw which rotates inside the bowl.

The sense of anticipation grows as the olives are delivered to the processing plant, unloaded into receiving the hoppers, passed through strippers to remove any impurities, and then washed and drained before processing. They are then crushed, turned in malaxers, and spun in high-speed centrifuges to separate out the olive oil.

At last, the 'liquid gold' begins to pour into the final vessel. It is at this point that a tasting cup is eased into the stream for the first sample of the season's olive-appreciated oil.

As the cup is lifted, there is a pause whilst the fresh aroma that wafts through the air is appreciated. This gives the first indication of the level of fruitiness. The olive oil is then sipped, coat the inside of the palates with viscous oil to assess the taste – is it bitter or mild? The greater the bitterness, the higher the level of antioxidants. When swallowed, is there the characteristic 'bite' or pepperiness in the back of the throat, an indication of the oil's pungency, also a level of antioxidant polyphenols.

The time between harvest and pulping does not exceed 24 hours. Morocco Gold extra virgin olive oil is unfiltered to retain all of its natural properties and goodness. Nothing is added or taken away so that it is the result of the soil, the sun, and the rain only.

It is an incredibly rewarding and enriching experience to know when harvesting is underway and that the new harvest of Morocco Gold will shortly be available. It is also incredibly rewarding to be part of a wholly natural process that has lasted for centuries.

Every aspect of olive production ultimately affects the oil itself: the growing region (climate, altitude, soil character), methods of growing, harvesting, and transporting the fruit, as well as extraction and storage methods. The care that is taken in each of these steps not only affects the taste and quality of the olive oil but its cost, yield, and shelf life.

Morocco Gold Olive Harvesters: The Sisterhood

Morocco's agricultural sector employs approximately 40% of the nation's workforce, nearly half of whom are women. Participating in local farming empowers Moroccan women, giving them influence over household income and expenditures. These jobs help to reduce rural poverty at least twice as effectively as other initiatives, both raising household incomes and lowering food costs.

Morocco Gold works with a co-operative that provides local women with business and educational opportunities. The group, which also grows almonds and walnuts, extracts, and sells oils locally and regionally. With the revenue earned from these endeavors, many members are able to pay for their children's education and help fund community infrastructure in remote villages, slowing rural de-population into cities like Fez and Marrakech.

At the end of a busy harvesting day, these harvesters return home to sip mint tea with their families. They share khobz, a typical round loaf cooked in a wood oven, paired with garlic scented green and black olives. The ingredients these women use to make traditional dishes like bessara - fave bean soup with olive oil, cumin, and paprika - come from nearby, sometimes from their own gardens.

Environment & Sustainability

Care of the environment is at the heart of the farming methods used. Even the left-over paste after pressing the olives is turned into briquettes for domestic fuel in rural areas. This reduces cutting down trees for firewood, and so prevents soil erosion.

In 2019 it was reported that British supermarkets admitted that they could be selling olive oil produced in a way that kills millions of songbirds every year. Many harvesters across Italy, Spain, and France suck olives from trees using machines and do this at night, which means sleeping birds who think they have found sanctuary in the olive branches are dazzled by the bright lights and sucked to their deaths. Harvesting in this way is done during the evening as it is believed to preserve the aroma of the olives, due to the cooler air temperatures. (10)

Birds including robins, goldfinches, greenfinches, warblers, and wagtails are among the worst affected during the harvest season. Findings in the journal Nature suggested that over two million birds were killed in Spain alone in a year.

The gorgeously picturesque area in the foothills of the Atlas Mountains where we source our fabulous extra virgin olive oil is hilly, and the distribution of the olive trees preclude the use of the types of mechanized harvesting machinery that has caused such concern. All the olives that go into Morocco Gold are hand-picked.

Extra Virgin Olive Oil, Health, And The Environment

We created Morocco Gold extra virgin olive oil for health-conscious, discerning food lovers across all cultures and culinary backgrounds. When we speak with our customers at our tasting events they always ask about our source in the foothills of the Atlas Mountains as well as how it is produced. They care passionately about the taste, how high-quality extra virgin olive oil like Morocco Gold has proven health benefits and increase the impact on the environment.

We were therefore fascinated with a new study by researchers from the University of Oxford and the University of Minnesota that demonstrates foods that are considered to be healthy, such as whole-grain cereals, fruits, vegetables, legumes, nuts, and *olive oil*, also have the lowest environmental impact.

This extensive research by Michael A Clark, Marco Springmann, Jason Hill, and David Tilman, published in the journal Proceedings of the National Academy of Sciences (PNAS) (11) shows that eating healthier also means eating more sustainably and reveals a clear link between healthy food and environmental sustainability.

Food choices are shifting globally in ways that are negatively affecting both human health and the environment. Here the researchers considered how consuming an additional serving per day of each of 15 foods key food groups is associated with 5 health outcomes in adults and 5 aspects of agriculturally driven environmental degradation.

The researchers found that "while there is substantial variation in the health outcomes of different foods, foods associated with a larger reduction in disease risk for one health outcome are often associated with larger reductions in disease risk for other health outcomes. Likewise, foods with lower impacts on one metric of environmental harm tend to have lower impacts on others".

"Additionally, of the foods associated with improved health (whole grain cereals, fruits, vegetables, legumes, nuts, *olive oil*, and fish), all except fish have among the *lowest environmental impacts*, and fish has markedly lower impacts than red meats and processed moats. Foods associated with the largest negative environmental impacts—unprocessed and processed red meat—are consistently associated with the largest increases in disease risk.

Thus, dietary transitions toward greater consumption of healthier foods would generally improve environmental sustainability, although processed foods high in sugars harm health but can have relatively low environmental impacts. These findings could help consumers, policy makers, and food companies to better understand the multiple health and environmental implications of food choices".

As part of the study, the researchers examined the impact of consuming an additional serving per day of fifteen specific foods on five "health outcomes" in adults that are brought on by poor diets and account for nearly 40 percent of global mortality, specifically: mortality, type two diabetes, stroke, coronary heart disease, and colorectal cancer.

At the same time, the effects on five "aspects of agriculturally driven environmental degradation" were studied, including greenhouse gas emissions, land use, water use, acidification, and eutrophication (the last two are forms of nutrient pollution).

The foods included chicken, dairy, eggs, fish, fruits, legumes, nuts, *olive oil,* potatoes, processed red meat, refined grain cereals, sugar-sweetened beverages, unprocessed red meat, vegetables, and whole-grain cereals.

By comparing the five health and five environmental impacts of each food, the researchers determined that foods with the lowest environmental impacts often have the largest health benefits. Foods such as whole-grain cereals, fruits, vegetables, legumes, nuts, *olive oil*, and fish had the most positive impact on health while also having the lowest environmental impact (with the exception of fish).

Conversely, the foods with the largest environmental impacts, such as unprocessed and processed red meat, were also associated with the highest risk of disease. Minimally processed, health-boosting plant foods and olive oil were found to have a low environmental impact, but so did processed foods high in sugar that are harmful to health, such as sugar-sweetened beverages.

Where Morocco Gold Fits In

What we set out to achieve was to: promote Morocco as an undiscovered source of high quality extra virgin olive oil; support healthy eating and lifestyle choices through all-natural, genuine, high quality extra virgin olive oil; set a new standard for provenance, authenticity, and the guarantee of extra virgin quality; educate consumers about olive oil as an original 'superfood,' rich in health enhancing polyphenols; help to transform the olive oil sector in Morocco and bring this centuries-old 'superfood' to international customers.

Morocco Gold is a natural, unfiltered, ultra-premium, polyphenol rich extra virgin olive oil. It's exquisite taste and health enhancing qualities are guaranteed by our rigorous testing, provenance and authenticity, and strict adherence to single sourcing, with no blending or mixing.

Sustainability and care for the environment is carried forward into our carefully designed bottle and packaging, which are fully re-cyclable with no waste.

As consumers in the UK and other markets are showing greater interest in healthy eating, lifestyles, and wider wellbeing, provenance authenticity and high quality have become paramount.

Testing For Quality: Extra Virgin Olive Oil Analysis Explained

International trade standards specify that extra virgin olive oil is extracted exclusively from olives, solely by mechanical means, without excessive heating or any chemical processing. Extra virgin olive oil is a natural product that does not need much to be preserved. It contains antioxidants, Nature's preservatives that extend the oil's shelf life if stored in a sealed bottle, away from the light and in cool temperature. Compared to wine making, extra virgin olive oil production is a simpler and faster process. But unlike wine, olive oil does not improve with age. It is at its best when fresh but will unavoidably change over time. Yet the volatile components that give extra virgin olive oil like Morocco Gold its desirable "green notes", the flavour and aroma that consumer and tasters desire, will eventually disappear over time.

Three basic laboratory assays are required to determine the oil's grade. They measure olive oil's attributes related to quality of the olive fruit and its processing and assess the oil's present state.

From Olive Fruit To Bottled Oil

Superior extra virgin olive oil like Morocco Gold is obtained only when harvest, milling, and processing of olives are properly managed. Along those steps, there are two naturally occurring and interrelated processes that must be understood as they impact the olive oil's quality: lipolysis and oxidation. Lipolysis (a form of hydrolysis) begins on the olive fruit as it ripens and is caused by enzymes present in the fruit, which are later on removed with the vegetation water. Lipolytic enzymes break down major olive oil components and generate free fatty acids, precursors to olive oil change of condition.

Oxidation (more specifically, auto-oxidation) is triggered when the oil enters in contact with oxygen in the air, first during the milling process and later on during storage in tanks and bottles. Oxidation produces peroxides from some fatty acids. Peroxides are unstable compounds that are further oxidized to yield volatile and non-volatile components that give rise to off-flavours and undesirable aromas in the oil (secondary oxidation). The other form of oxidation, photo oxidation, is usually minor and negligible if the oil is stored in the dark. In brief: lipolysis generates free fatty acids, and oxidation causes the formation of peroxides from these fatty acids (primary oxidation), eventually leading to rancidity and degradation of the oil over time (secondary oxidation).

Attaining extra virgin olive oil of superior quality requires minimizing the generation of free fatty acids by hydrolysis and delaying the onset of oxidation. The oxidation process in extra virgin olive oil takes place in three stages: initiation, propagation, and termination.

Figure 1: Olive Oil Oxidation

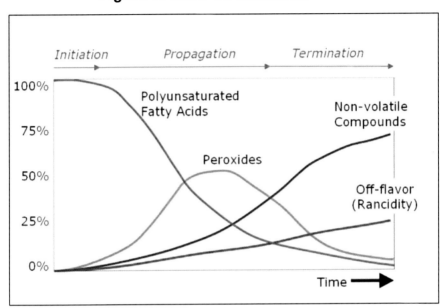

Figure 1 shows how the oxidation of fatty acids in olive oil changes with time. Once the oil has been decanted or contrifuged, the free fatty acid level (or free acidity) will gradually decline while the oil remains in ctorage [Declining free acidity is represented in the graph by the down-sloping line from upper-left to lower-right.] During the initiation stage, free fatty acids present in the oil become slowly oxidized, giving rise to small amounts of peroxides. Since peroxides, in turn, decompose into other substances, the overall peroxide level does not increase rapidly. However, when certain levels of peroxides are reached in the oil, a propagation stage ensues during which peroxide levels will rapidly increase, as peroxides beget other peroxides. [Increasing accumulation of peroxides is represented in the graph by the rising left-side of the curve.] During the termination stage, peroxides further decompose, giving off numerous off-flavour compounds that humans can detect, even if present at extremely low concentrations—below parts per million. Therefore, even when just a tiny fraction of peroxides degrades into undesirable compounds, the oil will begin to taste rancid. [Rancidity is represented by the lower line rising from the bottom-left to the right of the graph.]

If the quality of the olive fruit was very good and free acidity levels were low when processing the olives, there may be a time lag of up to 3 years before peroxide levels in the oil become problematic (that is, the initiation period is long). But if the olive fruit was spoiled, the temperature during processing was too high, or the malaxation time too long, there is an increased risk of reaching higher peroxide levels much sooner, thereby shortening the oil's shelf life. [Peroxides' evolution is represented by the bell-shaped curve in the centre of the graph.]

Olive Oil Quality Attributes

The basic olive oil parameters measured analytically are Free Fatty Acids (FFA), Peroxide Value (PV), and UV absorbance. In combination, they will indicate proper or inadequate handling of the olive fruit prior to milling and assess the oil's present state of oxidation.

Free Fatty Acids (FFA) or Free Acidity

As mentioned earlier, free fatty acid formation precedes most, if not all, oil deterioration. Free acidity levels increase by hydrolysis of the major oil molecules in the fruit (triglycerides) early in the production process, from harvest through milling, while water and plant enzymes are still in contact with the oil. For this reason, milling the olives soon after harvest, and promptly separating oil from vegetation water is critical to maintaining a low initial free acidity level, essential for higher-quality oil.

Free acidity values provide an indication of how the fruit was handled prior to processing and the length of time from harvest to milling. Free acidity is also an early indicator of the potential longevity of the oil. Higher quality oils recently produced will exhibit very low acidity—it may be no higher than 0.35% in the best extra virgin olive oils like Morocco Gold.

Peroxide Value (PV)

Peroxides, which are flavourless, are generated from the oxidation of polyunsaturated fatty acids in the oil (linoleic and linolenic acids). Peroxides are unstable, usually building up slowly and eventually leading to oil rancidity. The onset of this decay process may be delayed for up to 3 years in good extra virgin olive oil, rich in radical-scavenging antioxidants. But once peroxides are present, rancidity is unavoidable. Peroxide Value identifies the early stages of oxidation. Subsequent oxidation is detected through UV absorbance and by the oil's sensory properties, which result from the peroxides' breakdown.

To reduce peroxide levels and therefore delay oxidation of high peroxide oils, blending may be a viable recourse. Otherwise, refining is the only option to eliminate peroxides and remove off-flavour substances. Obviously, the resulting product will not be extra virgin olive oil.

Ultraviolet (UV) Absorbance

UV tests determine the ultraviolet light absorbance measured by shining UV light through the oil at several specific wavelengths. Absorbance at K232 nm (nanometers), K270 nm, and Delta K correlate with the state of oxidation by detecting specific oxidized compounds, some generated from secondary oxidation, and also detecting possible adulteration with refined oils.

Interpreting Analysis Results

The standard set of quality tests for grading olive oil includes organoleptic (sensory) tests and the three basic analyses: FFA, PV, and UV. The International Olive

Committee's (IOC) olive oil standards specify the precise measurement thresholds to be met for oils to be graded as extra virgin, virgin, and so on. Whenever analytical parameters (FFA, PV, and UV) exceed a given threshold, the oil is classified as the next lower quality grade. But experts agree that a quality extra virgin olive oil can meet more stringent thresholds than the standard, reflecting the freshness and quality of truly superior oil. The standard FFA threshold is 0.8% acidity, but fresh, high-quality extra virgin olive oil can certainly achieve FFA values of 0.3 % or lower.

Peroxide Values vary widely over time. Some oils may meet the extra virgin olive oil's 20 mq/kg threshold while already showing early signs of rancidity. Experience indicates that high-quality, recently milled oils exhibit peroxide values below 12 mq/kg. Truly excellent oils may have PV as low as 7 mq/kg (9 mq/kg for organic oil). The lower the PV, the more likely the oil's shelf life will be extended.

Regarding UV absorbance, though the standards call for K232 below 2.5 and K270 below 0.22, superior olive oil will exhibit K232 values below 1.85 (2 for organic oil) and K270 below 0.17. As mentioned before, low values correlate with high-quality oil, as UV absorbance detects early and later states of oxidation.

Conclusion

A basic set of analysis provides producers and buyers and ultimately customers with valuable information about the quality of fruit and processing that went into the extra virgin olive oil. That is why we have included the results of our own analysis on each and every bottle of Morocco Gold extra virgin olive oil.

CHAPTER 3.
WHAT MAKES MOROCCO GOLD SO SPECIAL: POLYPHENOLS

Why Choose Extra Virgin Olive Oil?

There are many reasons why people choose extra virgin olive oil like Morocco Gold over other types of oils. Whether this is extra virgin olive oil as part of a healthy diet, extra virgin olive oil for its delicious taste, or extra virgin oil because of its now well-researched and documented health benefits. Extra virgin olive oil is probably the most extensively researched foodstuff on the planet, and the health benefits are evidence based.

What Makes Extra Virgin Olive Oil So Healthy?

Extra virgin olive oil, sunflower oil, and canola oil are high in monounsaturated fat (the healthy-for-you kind of fat). So, what would put extra virgin olive oil above the others if their fat make-up so similar? It's not just about the kind of fat molecules that they are made up of, extra virgin olive oil has some extra magic. The biggest thing that makes extra virgin olive oil so healthy is its unique disease-fighting component.

Thanks to the recent spotlight on the Mediterranean Diet, extensive research has been done on the phytonutrient composition of olive oil. What has been discovered is an extensive list of phytonutrients; one of the most praised is its polyphenols. The number of polyphenols found in extra virgin olive oil is truly amazing!

What Are Polyphenols?

Many of the fruits and vegetables we consume contain large numbers of compounds critical for life. One such type of compound is known as antioxidants. Polyphenols are powerful antioxidants.

Polyphenols are a group of over 500 phytochemicals, which are naturally occurring micronutrients in plants. These compounds give a plant its colour and can help to protect it from various dangers. When you eat plants with polyphenols, you reap the health benefits as well. Polyphenols are a key component in extra virgin olive oil and are considered to be one of the best health enhancing benefits within the oil

Why are antioxidants so important for our health? Oxidation is a natural process our cells use to create energy from the oxygen we inhale. As energy is being produced in our cells, some oxygen molecules (known as oxygen free radicals or reactive oxygen species) are produced as a by-product of these processes. These oxygen free radicals can damage your cells and DNA when in high concentration. Continuous damage by oxygen free radicals most often termed oxidative stress can lead to various conditions including:

Various forms of cancer

Cardiovascular disease

Diabetes

Osteoporosis

Alzheimer's Disease

Dementia

Wrinkles associated with age

Unfortunately, the production of these harmful chemicals is sometimes enhanced by the environment we live in. Several lifestyle, stress, and environmental factors shown to increase the production of oxygen free radicals include (but are not limited to):

Cigarette smoke

Alcohol consumption

High blood sugar levels

Air pollution

High intake of polyunsaturated fats

Excessive ultraviolet radiation exposure

Various bacterial or viral infections

Antioxidant deficiency

So how do antioxidants fit into the grand scheme of our bodies and our health? Antioxidants are chemicals known to be 'molecular scavengers' that help neutralize oxygen free radicals, thus preventing oxidative stress from occurring. There are hundreds of known antioxidants, some of which we consume in our daily diets:

Vitamin A

Vitamin C

Vitamin E

Selenium

Manganese

Carotenoids

And....POLYPHENOLS

It's also thought that polyphenols contribute to keeping the body being in an anti-inflammatory state. This is also associated with a lower risk of several chronic diseases.

They also protect the olive oil from oxidative damage and contribute to its superior longevity and shelf life. They also affect the taste of extra virgin olive oil and give it its distinctive bitter flavour.

Polyphenols In Morocco Gold Extra Virgin Olive Oil

The high polyphenol content of Morocco Gold extra virgin olive oil is dependent on three factors. First is the variety of the olive, secondly the climate and terroir of the growing region, and thirdly the actual time in the growing season that the crop is harvested.

Morocco Gold is pressed from the Picholine Marocaine, the only type of olive to go into Morocco Gold. Oil from this variety is renowned for its high polyphenol count, oxidative stability, and longevity.

Our olives are grown in a valley that is about 2,000 feet above sea level. This helps to create the additional climatic challenges that encourage polyphenol uptake within the olive tree. It is also an area with naturally occurring high phenols in the soil itself.

In soils, phenols are released over an extended period of time from decomposing plant materials. This causes complex organic compounds to be slowly oxidized or to break down into simpler forms of sugars, amino sugars, aliphatic and phenolic organic acids. These are further transformed into microbial biomass or are reorganized, and further oxidized, into humic assemblages (fulvic and humic acids), which bind to clay minerals.

There has been a long debate about the ability of plants to uptake humic substances through their root systems and to metabolize them. There is now a consensus about how humus plays a hormonal role rather than simply a nutritional role in plant physiology. Olive trees grown in 'challenging' conditions encourage the uptake of naturally occurring phenols in the soil. This in turn, aids the circulatory system within the olive tree, with the phenols eventually finding their way to the olive fruit itself.

Thirdly, our olives are picked when the fruit is young and green. As the olives age on the tree, the colour of the olive changes to red and then black, the size of the olive increases, thus producing more oil, but the polyphenol level decreases. There is a great deal of expertise within the farming community where we source our oil to ensure that the harvest is collected at the optimum time to maximise the polyphenol level.

Extraction Process For Extra Virgin Olive Oil

"The release of phenols and the formation of volatiles are two basic components of virgin olive oil quality that directly relate to the mechanical extraction process itself. In this ambit, control of endogenous enzymes of olive fruit during processing is the most critical point in the mechanical extraction process of olive oil. In fact, the secoiridoid concentration in the virgin olive oil is largely due to the activation of the glycosidases of olive fruit that activate the formation of aglycon, while the oxidoreductases such as polyphenol-oxidase (PPO) and peroxidase (POD) can catalyse their oxidation during the oil mechanical extraction process and subsequently trigger the autoxidation mechanism". (12)

So, what does all this mean? The types of polyphenol present in extra virgin olive oil are influenced by the extraction/pressing process. To be extra virgin olive oil, the extraction needs to be done solely by mechanical means and at low temperatures. This has a direct effect on the resulting polyphenol content. There also must be no mixing or blending with other oils and no chemical additives. This is how the natural goodness and health enriching qualities of the extra virgin olive oil is preserved.

The Polyphenols Present In Morocco Gold extra virgin olive oil are:

3,4 DHPEA-EDA

Hydroxytyrosol

Lignanes

Ligstroside aglycone (p, HPEA-EA)

Oleuropein aglycone (3,4 DHPEA-EA)

Oleocanthal (p, HPEA-EDA)

Tyrosol

The following illustrates the range of chronic conditions where research into these polyphenols oil has demonstrated positive effects.

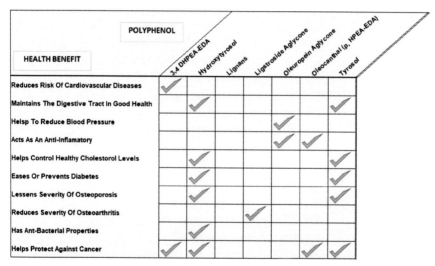

HEALTH BENEFIT	3,4 DHPEA-EDA	Hydroxytyrosol	Lignans	Ligstroside Aglycone	Oleuropein Aglycone	Oleocanthal (p, HPEA-EDA)	Tyrosol
Reduces Risk Of Cardiovascular Diseases	✓						
Maintains The Digestive Tract In Good Health		✓					✓
Helsp To Reduce Blood Pressure				✓			
Acts As An Anti-Inflamatory				✓	✓		
Helps Control Healthy Cholestorol Levels		✓					✓
Eases Or Prevents Diabetes		✓					✓
Lessens Severity Of Osteoporosis		✓					✓
Reduces Severity Of Osteoarthritis			✓				
Has Ant-Bacterial Properties		✓					
Helps Protect Against Cancer	✓	✓				✓	✓

In fact, the European Food Safety Authority has now approved health claims for extra virgin olive oils with a polyphenol content of more than 250 mg/kg. Morocco Gold contains polyphenols well above this level.

Healthy Compounds In Extra Virgin Olive Oil Still Present After Exposure To Heat

New research confirms the key components in extra virgin olive oil survive temperature. The healthiest compounds found in extra virgin olive oil do not disappear when the oil is used for cooking, according to new research published in the scientific journal, Antioxidants. The implication may have an impact on future nutritional guidelines.

Researchers from the University of Barcelona focused on evaluating how the attributes of olive oil change when it is used for sautéing in a household kitchen. After cooking at a moderate temperature, (polyphenols and antioxidants) were still in the oil and in concentrations high enough to meet the E.U. parameters, meaning this oil should be used for cooking. *Julián Lozano Castellón, project coordinator*

Polyphenol: 3,4 DHPEA-EDA

3,4-DHPEA-EDA is a polyphenol in the family of Tyrosols. It is synonymous with 3,4-DHPEA-Elenolic acid Di-Aldehyde and Oleuropein-aglycone di-aldehyde. Its chemical formula is: $C_{17}H_{20}O_6$

What This Polyphenol Does: It's Role In Health Benefits

Diets in which fat is significantly provided by extra virgin olive oil have been associated with a low incidence of cardiovascular diseases. In this study, the anti-inflammatory effect of 3,4-DHPEA-EDA on the endothelium was examined.

The study was based on the production of the pro-inflammatory chemokine CCL2, following in vitro stimulation of primary human endothelial cells. The study found that pre-treatment of cells with 3,4-DHPEA-EDA resulted in inhibition of CCL2 secretion.

Why is this so important?

The Endothelium, Blood Vessels, and Endothelial Cells

Almost all tissues depend on a blood supply, and the blood supply depends on endothelial cells which form the linings of the blood vessels. Endothelial cells have a remarkable capacity to adjust their number and arrangement to suit local requirements. They create an adaptable life-support system, extending by cell migration into almost every region of the body.

Endothelial cells form the barrier between vessels and tissues. They control the flow of substances and fluid into and out of a tissue. An impaired function can lead to serious health issues throughout the body. Endothelial cells line blood vessels and lymphatic vessels, they are found exclusively in vascularized tissue.

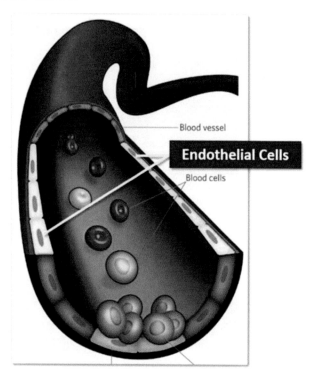

Endothelial cells are nearly ubiquitous throughout the body. If it were not for endothelial cells extending and remodelling the network of blood vessels, tissue growth and repair would be impossible.

However, there are two major instances where dysfunction of endothelial cells is involved in pathogenesis of a medical condition. First, in coronary artery disease, endothelial cells are damaged. So, the generation of new vascular cells to restore organ function following a myocardial infarction is of high research interest. Another example is atherosclerosis, where endothelial dysfunction arising from chronic inflammation within the arterial wall causes a pathological change of blood vessels.

The effect of 3,4-DHPEA-EDA on CCL2 expression was observed at the transcriptional level. Functional data have shown that 3,4-DHPEA-EDA diminished monocyte adhesion to HUVECs (human umbilical vein endothelial cells are cells derived from the endothelium of veins from the umbilical cord. They are used as a laboratory model system for the study of the function and pathology of endothelial cells). These results point on the use of 3,4- DHPEA-EDA as a novel drug aimed to prevent or reduce inflammation of endothelium. (13)

Endothelial Cells And Cancer

Cancerous tissue is as dependent on a blood supply as is normal tissue, and this has led to a surge of interest in endothelial cell biology. It is hoped that by blocking the formation of new blood vessels through drugs that act on endothelial cells, it may be possible to block the growth of cancerous tumours.

Polyphenol: Hydroxytyrosol

Hydroxytyrosol is a powerful polyphenol that occurs naturally in the olive fruit, pulp, leaves, and mill waste waters. Chemically, hydroxytyrosol is described as 4-(2-hydroxyethyl)-1,2-benzendiol, with the chemical formula $C_8H_{10}O_3$.[2]

Hydroxytyrosol is a well-known minor component found in extra virgin olive oil, which is derived from hydrolysis of the polyphenol oleuropein during olive maturation and olive oil storage. The compound plays an important role in the complex and varied flavour of olives and olive oil. It is also a vital component which largely adds to the stability and longevity of extra virgin olive oil.

Hydroxytyrosol is hydrophilic and is absorbed in a dose-dependent manner in humans, with absorption occurring in the small intestine and colon. Uniquely, hydroxytyrosol is the only polyphenol that is able to cross the blood brain barrier, which allows it to have a significant action to scavenge free radicals in the nervous system. (14)

Health Benefits Of Hydroxytyrosol In Extra Virgin Olive Oil

Hydroxytyrosol has a potent antioxidant activity. It has one of the highest known ORAC (oxygen radical absorbance capacity) results known for a natural antioxidant. ORAC is a method used to determine the antioxidant capacity of a food or chemical substance. There is also evidence related to the health benefits of hydroxytyrosol in extra virgin olive oil in the following areas:

Anticancer Activity

Hydroxytyrosol in extra virgin olive oil has the capacity to inhibit proliferation and promote apoptosis of several tumour cells. Therefore, it has been suggested that hydroxytyrosol may have anticancer effects. The exact mechanism of these effects is not well defined, and research continues in this space.

Anti-inflammatory Activity

Research has shown that hydroxytyrosol in extra virgin olive oil can reduce the production of cytokine tumour necrosis factor-alpha (TNF alpha) in animal models of inflammation. Animal based research has also shown that hydroxytyrosol in extra virgin olive oil may be able to reduce acute inflammation and associated pain.

Antimicrobial Activity

In vitro experiments have shown that hydroxytyrosol in extra virgin olive oil has antimicrobial properties against infectious respiratory and gastrointestinal pathogens. It is also known that hydroxytyrosol in extra virgin olive oil has activity against gram-positive and gram-negative bacteria. In general, polyphenols have been reported to have wide antimicrobial activity, such as antibacterial, antiviral, and antifungal effects.

Antithrombotic Activity

A human study showed that hydroxytyrosol in extra virgin olive oil was able to lower serum thromboxane B2 levels, leading to an anti-aggregatory platelet effect. Other research supports this finding, showing that hydroxytyrosol significantly reduces platelet aggregation.

Antiatherogenic Capacity And Cardioprotective Effect

It is known that hydroxytyrosol in extra virgin olive oil is a powerful scavenger of free radicals, which allows for the reduction in oxidation of low-density-lipoproteins (LDL), potentially reducing the risk of atherosclerosis.

Retino-Protective Activity

Hydroxytyrosol in extra virgin olive oil may play a role in reducing the risk of age-related macular degeneration however further research is required in this area to determine the exact mechanism and importance of this preliminary research finding.

Skin Related Effects

It is believed that oxidative stress plays a major role in UVA-induced protein damage to the skin. Preliminary research shows that hydroxytyrosol in extra virgin olive oil can work to prevent such UVA damage in melanoma cells.

Lignans: A Major Polyphenol Found In Extra Virgin Olive Oil

Because extra virgin olive oil is an important component of the Mediterranean diet, increasing levels of research have been carried out to determine the source of the health benefits associated with extra virgin olive oil, in particular the major antioxidant polyphenols it contains. Structural analysis includes spectroscopic techniques, including mass spectrometry and nuclear magnetic resonance (NMR) testing.

Lignans are polyphenols that accumulate in the woody tissues, seeds, and roots of many plants, including olives. These molecules are thought to be directly involved in the defence mechanisms of plants and now have been found to be useful for humans. Foods containing high amounts of lignan precursors have been found to be protective against breast, colon, and prostate cancer.

These lignans, which are potent antioxidants, are absent in seed oils and virtually absent in refined virgin oils. As with other polyphenols, there is considerable variation in lignan concentrations in different varieties of olive. (15)

New Research: Extra Virgin Olive Oil And Reductions In Breast Cancer Risk

Javier Menendez from the Catalan Institute of Oncology and Antonio Segura-Carretero from the University of Granada in Spain led a team of researchers who set out to investigate which parts of olive oil were most active against cancer.

Menendez said, "Our findings reveal for the first time that all the major complex phenols present in extra-virgin olive oil drastically suppress overexpression of the cancer gene HER2 in human breast cancer cells".

Extra virgin olive oil is the oil that results from pressing olives without the use of heat or chemical treatments. It contains phytochemicals that are otherwise lost in the refining process. Menendez and colleagues separated the oil into fractions and tested these against breast cancer cells in lab experiments. All the fractions containing the major extra virgin phytochemical polyphenols (lignans and secoiridoids) were found to effectively inhibit HER2.

Although these findings provide new insights on the mechanisms by which good quality extra virgin olive oil rich in polyphenols might contribute to a lowering of breast cancer risk in a HER2-dependent manner, extreme caution must be applied when applying the lab results to the human situation. As the authors point out, "The active phytochemicals (i.e. lignans and secoiridoids) exhibited tumoricidal effects against cultured breast cancer cells at concentrations that are unlikely to be achieved in real life by consuming olive oil".

Nevertheless, and according to the authors, "These findings, together with the fact that humans have safely been ingesting significant amounts of lignans and secoiridoids as long as they have been consuming olives and extra-virgin oil, strongly suggest that these polyphenols might provide an excellent and safe platform for the design of new anti-breast-cancer drugs". (16)

Polyphenol: Ligstroside-Aglycone (LA)

This polyphenol is synonymous with p-HPEA-Elenolic acid. It is a member of the Tyrosol family of polyphenols and has the chemical formula: $C_{19}H_{22}O_7$

While the information on LA bioactivity is limited, a few years ago, LA was demonstrated to behave as an antioxidant. Furthermore, LA has been shown to have anti-inflammatory effects by controlling and downregulating NF-κB (NF-kB is a type of DNA that is thought to play a pivotal role in the initiation of osteoarthritis and the perpetuation of chronic inflammation in rheumatoid arthritis) as well as the potential to induce a caloric restriction-like state that affects the muscle, brain, fat tissue and kidney, particularly through activation and increased levels of sirtuins. (Sirtuins are a family of proteins that regulate cellular health. They play a key role in regulating cellular homeostasis, keeping cells in balance).

A Study Of Ligstroside-Aglycone In Treatment Of Osteoarthritis

In a recent study at the Faculty Of Pharmacy Seville and the Biomedical Research Institute Coruna (M.S. Meiss, M. Sanchez-Hidalgo, A. Gonzales-Benjumea) the effectiveness of LA on osteoarthritis (OA) was examined. (17)

Osteoarthritis is currently, the most frequent cause of pain, deformity, and dysfunction in the elderly. It is a late-onset, complex disease of the joint, characterised by progressive failure of the extracellular cartilage matrix (ECM), together with changes in the synovium and subchondral bone.

OA persists as the most common form of arthritis worldwide and the sixth leading cause of disability. Unlike most tissues, articular cartilage does not contain blood vessels, nerves, or lymphatics, rather, articular cartilage is composed of a dense ECM with a sparse distribution of highly specialised cells called chondrocytes. Aberrant expression of degradative proteases or catabolic mediators is induced in OA chondrocytes that contribute to cartilage destruction.

To date, there is no definitive cure for this debilitating disease. The mechanism of disease progression in OA remains largely unknown, and thus, to date, a more personalised approach is required to aid patient disease management. Current treatments are targeted at reducing symptoms of the inflammatory reaction that occurs following the destruction of the essential joint cartilage. These treatments, however, do not prevent the significant pain associated with OA or the often-reported restriction of mobility and activity.

To address this unmet need, alternative approaches, including the use of polyphenols as a novel therapeutic intervention are under examination. The objective of this study was to analyse if the polyphenols found in extra virgin olive oil can reverse the catabolic activity that contributes to cartilage destruction in OA.

Two polyphenols from extra virgin olive oil, oleocanthal (OLC), and ligstroside aglycone (LA), plus a chemically modified acetylated ligstroside aglycone (A-LA), and two marine polyunsaturated fatty acids, eicosapentaenoic acid (EPA) and docosahexaenoic acid (DHA), were examined as potential anti-inflammatory agents for OA.

The Results

Acetylated ligstroside showed the most promising results for implementation in treating OA as it reduced the expression of pro-inflammatory genes such as inducible nitric oxide (*INOS*), matrix metalloprotease-13 (*MMP13*), and interleukin-1β (*IL1B*) at both RNA and protein levels; decreased nitric oxide (NO) levels from cartilage explants and also reduced proteoglycan (PG) losses in human osteoarthritic cartilage explants and chondrocytes.

These results substantiato the role of polyphenols in OA with implications for therapeutic intervention and our understanding of OA pathophysiology.

Recently, data from the Osteoarthritis Initiative (OAI) have demonstrated that adherence to the Mediterranean diet is associated not only with better quality of life but also, significantly, with a lower prevalence of OA. Given that the general population can be viewed as at risk in the development of OA in later life, an approach that relies on dietary modification is attractive in terms of risk/benefit and, potentially, an approach that is more likely to be implementable. Indeed, as an alternative to traditional treatments, alternative modalities have come to the fore, including the effects of polyphenols as non-invasive treatments, based on the evidence that epigenetic changes are triggered by dietary nutrients and contribute to the prevention of a number of diseases. (18)

Polyphenol: Oleuropein Aglycone (OA)

Oleuropein aglycone is a glycosylated Seco-iridoid, a type of bitter phenolic compound found in green olive skin, flesh, seeds, and leaves. The term oleuropein is derived from the botanical name of the olive tree, Olea Europaea. The chemical formula is: $C_{25}H_{32}O_{13}$.

Oleuropein aglycone is one of the chief polyphenols found in extra virgin olive oil. It is getting more and more global attention within the scientific and medical communities due to its biological properties including in anti-Alzheimer's disease, anti-breast cancer, anti-inflammatory, anti-hyperglycemic effect, and anti-oxidative properties.

OA is derived from the de-glycosylation of oleuropein that exists in the leaves and stones of the olive fruit during the maturation period and is obtained during the pressing of the olives.

A Study Of The Effect Of Oleuropein Aglycone On Amyloidosis & Associated Bowel Dysfunction

Amyloidosis is the name for a group of rare but serious condition caused by a build-up of an abnormal protein called amyloid in organs and tissues throughout the body. The build-up of amyloid protein deposits can make it difficult for the organs and tissues to work properly.

It had been reported that the aglycone form of oleuropein interferes with the build-up of a number of proteins associated with amyloidosis, particularly affecting neuro-degenerative diseases, preventing the growth of toxic oligomers (polymers with relatively few repeating units) and displaying protection against cognitive deterioration.

This study examined the relationships between the effects of OA on the aggregation and cell interactions of the D76N β2-microglobulin (D76N b2m) variant associated with a form of systemic amyloidosis leading to progressive bowel dysfunction at a cellular and biophysical level.

"The results indicated that OA protection against D76N b2m cytotoxicity results from a modification of the conformational and biophysical properties of its amyloid fibrils, also a modification of the cell bilayer surface properties of exposed cells.

The study showed that OA remodels not only D76N b2m aggregates but also the cell membrane interfering with the misfolded proteins-cell membrane association, in most cases an early event triggering amyloid–mediated cytotoxicity".

Or in simple terms, OA provides a protective barrier between health organ cells and harmful amyloid cells.

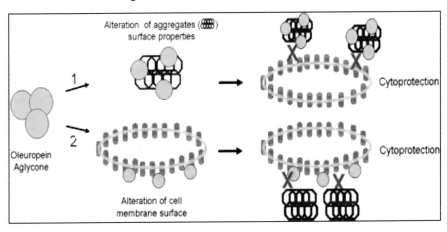

How oleuropein aglycone works to protect at a cellular level.

This confirms the polyphenol OA as a promising plant molecule useful against amyloid diseases. (19)

Other Biological Benefits Of Oleuropein Aglycone

Anti-Alzheimer's Disease Effect

Alzheimer's disease (AD) is a high social impact disease that represents approximately 55–60% of all dementias and affects 6% of the elderly. AD is marked by cognitive degradation with a progressive impact on daily living.

Amyloid β (Aβ) deposits and oligomers are found in AD. Recently reported findings to indicate that OA administration to mice can improve memory and behavioural performance by interfering with Aβ build-up. In addition, OA provides neuroprotection to cultured neuronal cells by preventing Aβ build-up, decreasing aggregate cytotoxicity, and counteracting related neuro-inflammation.

This suggests that OA administration could be regarded as a new way to prevent and cure AD.

Anti-Breast Cancer Effect

OA has been shown to be the most promising polyphenol in extra virgin olive oil in reducing breast cancer cell activity by suppressing the proliferation of Human Epidermal Growth Factor Receptor2 (HER2) breast carcinoma cells.

Anti-inflammatory Effect

Inflammation is a complex immune response to pathogens, damaged cells, or irritants and enables during infection or injury. Pain from inflammation is something most people experience at some point in their lives and a common daily occurrence for many people with arthritis. OA plays an anti-inflammatory role during chronic inflammation and improves tissue damage associated with collagen-induced arthritis.

In addition, OA may be responsible for inhibiting cyclooxygenase (COX) enzymes. COX is an enzyme that forms prostanoids, prostaglandins, prostacyclins, and thromboxanes, which are all contributors to the inflammatory response. Therefore, OA can play an effective role in anti-inflammatory activities.

Anti-Hyperglycemic Effect

Pancreatic amyloid deposits of amylin are characteristic indications of type II diabetes. OA has the ability to intervene with the early stages of build-up of these deposits and hinder the cellular damage they cause.

Anti-Oxidative Effect

Oxidation of low-density lipoproteins (LDL) is deemed to increase the incidence of atherogenesis, which is a potential cause of coronary heart disease. OA was reported to protect LDL in plasma against oxidation which is considered relevant in combating atherosclerotic disease. (20)

Polyphenol: p-HPEA-EDA (Oleocanthal)

p-HPEA-EDA, otherwise known as Oleocanthal, belongs to the Tyrosol family of polyphenols. It is the dialdehydic form of decarboxymethyl ligstroside aglycone. It is synonymous with p-HPEA-Elenolic acid Di-Aldohyde and Ligstroside-aglycone di-aldehyde. Its chemical formula is $C_{17}H_{20}O_5$

The Oleocanthal molecule is responsible for the peppery/stinging sensation at the back of your throat when you ingest certain extra virgin olive oils. In fact, this is how the molecule got its name, 'oleo' means oil, and 'canth' is Greek for stinging or prickly.

The importance and uniqueness of Oleocanthal in extra virgin olive oil is that it has strong antioxidant and anti-inflammatory properties. Its anti-inflammatory action on the body is very similar to ibuprofen, one of the non-steroidal anti-inflammatory drugs most widely consumed.

Non-steroidal anti-inflammatory drugs (NSAIDS) such as aspirin, paracetamol, and ibuprofen, can be differentiated from steroids because they have far fewer secondary effects. NSAIDS have proven to have very beneficial effects in diseases that involve chronic inflammation processes, such as degenerative and neurodegenerative illnesses (Alzheimer).

A Study On The Effect Of Oleocanthal In Extra Virgin Olive Oil On Cancer

Many studies have identified the components of extra virgin olive oil which confer health benefits, but few have tested the effect of high phenolic extra virgin olive oil on cancer. This is a gap that the research of Dr Limor Goren, who recently completed her PhD, and her colleagues at City University of New York set out to explore. (21)

The study explored the effects of oils containing varying levels of oleocanthal on anti-cancer effects. Dr Goren's study showed that extra virgin olive oil rich in oleocanthal is powerful enough to have an effect on cancer cells, while oleocanthal-poor olive oils do not.

The study has shown that oleocanthal specifically kills human cancer cells, but not normal, non-cancerous cells. The authors suggest that this is due to the ability of oleocanthal to induce the death of cancer cells through lysosomal membrane permeabilisation (LMP). (A lysosome is a membrane-bound cell organelle that contains digestive enzymes. Lysosomes are involved with various cell processes. They break down excess or worn-out cell parts. They may be used to destroy invading viruses and bacteria). Permeabilising the lysosomal membrane allows digestive enzymes stored inside this organelle to be released, which preferentially causes cell death in cancer cells.

Furthermore, recognizing that different olive oils have different oleocanthal concentrations due to their origin, harvest time, and processing methods, the researchers tested a variety of extra virgin olive oils to determine their respective concentrations of oleocanthal, which ranged from very low to very high.

The olive oils that had high oleocanthal content completely killed cancer cells in vitro (in a petri dish), in a manner similar to purified oleocanthal. The olive oils with average oleocanthal content reduced viability, but to a lesser extent. Those with no oleocanthal had no effect on cell viability.

Oleocanthal And Tumours In Mice

In addition, Dr Goren and colleagues also found that injection of oleocanthal into mice engineered to develop pancreatic neuroendocrine tumours, reduced their tumour burden and extended the lifespan of the mice. More specifically, the oleocanthal injections extended the lives of the mice by an average of four weeks. Based on lifespan conversion, if oleocanthal has the same effect in humans, it might extend human life by more than 10 years.

How Much Should Be Taken?

In order that oleocanthal may have protective effects on our health, like the rest of extra virgin olive oil polyphenols, daily and regular consumption is recommended. Four daily tablespoons of an extra virgin olive oil rich in Oleocanthal is equivalent to a consumption of 125 mg of ibuprofen, which would be, according to the researchers of the Andalusian society of Oleocanthal, a good basis to prevent or relieve chronic inflammatory processes and reduce the risks of cancer.

Tyrosol: A Key Polyphenol In Morocco Gold Extra Virgin Olive Oil

Tyrosol is a phenylethanoid, a derivative of phenethyl alcohol. It is a natural phenolic antioxidant present in a variety of natural sources. The principal source for the human diet is high quality extra virgin olive oil like Morocco Gold. As an antioxidant, tyrosol can protect cells against injury due to oxidation.

Along with hydroxytyrosol, tyrosol is one of the most abundant polyphenols in extra virgin olive oil, where they occur as such or in the form of esters of elenolic acid. There is an increasing level of research into these polyphenols and their properties to determine which is the most significant contributor towards the range of health benefits associated with high quality extra virgin olive oil.

Tyrosol is a colourless solid at room temperature, melting at 91–92°C, and slightly soluble in water. Hydroxytyrosol, on the other hand, appears as a clear colourless liquid at room temperature. It is now believed that this affects the rate of 'uptake' when ingested with hydoxytyrosol acting more quickly in the gut however tyrosol accumulating intercellularly over time to provide longer term protection due to its higher concentration and good bioavailability. (22)

Health Benefits Of Tyrosol

Its beneficial properties for human health are strongly related to the ability of the molecule to scavenge free radicals and reactive oxygen/nitrogen species as well as to activate endogenous antioxidant systems in the body.

CHAPTER 4.
EXTRA VIRGIN OLIVE OIL AND WELLNESS

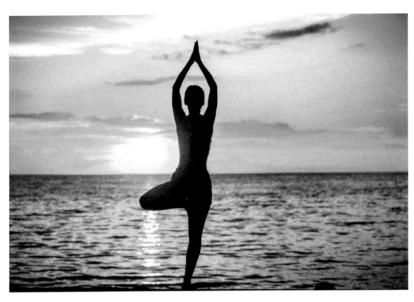

For many of us in 2021, our wellness routines, like so many facets of life, were completely overturned by Covid. We cancelled our restorative vacations and postponed our plans for wellness retreats. We started working from home and adjusted our social interactions.

Now for many of us, 2022 is about regaining what we lost and finding new ways to take care of ourselves. So, as we pick ourselves up, here is a simple lifestyle adjustment that is so easy to make that has the potential to add to our wellness experiences and change the way we approach our physical and emotional wellbeing.

Extra Virgin Olive Oil: Ancient Wisdom That Lives On

The olive is among the oldest known cultivated trees in the world - being grown before written language was invented.

Extra virgin olive oil is **the original** superfood. Its flavour and health enriching properties have been celebrated and enjoyed for centuries.

Olive oil has long been considered sacred. The olive branch was often a symbol of abundance, glory, and peace. Over the years, the olive has also been used to symbolize wisdom, fertility, power, and purity.

Olive oil was used for not only food and cooking, but also lighting, sacrificial offerings, ointment, and ceremonial anointment for priestly or royal office. The leafy branches of the olive tree were ritually offered to deities and powerful figures as emblems of benediction and purification, and they were used to crown the victors of friendly games and bloody wars.

Legend has it that Poseidon, the sea god, and Athena, goddess of wisdom, competed to find the gift that would be most valuable to humankind. Poseidon offered the horse and Athena the olive tree. Because of its many uses, the provision of heat, food, medicine, and perfume, the olive tree was chosen as the most valuable, and in return for Athena's contribution, the most powerful city in Greece was named Athens in her honour.

Is Olive Oil A Food Or A Medicine?

In Rome, olive oil was used for nearly everything in relation to their health. Roman medicine takes heavily from Greek doctors, who influenced European medicine for centuries, and Hippocrates, the father of modern medicine writes about over 60 different conditions or ailments that can be treated with olive oil, including skin problems, burns and wounds, ear infections, gynaecological problems, healing surgical scars, and much more. Many of these uses are still valid and are used as home remedies today.

"Let food be thy medicine and medicine be thy food"

Hippocrates: father of modern medicine

Olive oil was believed to bestow strength and youth, not least because of the tree's longevity and its tremendous resilience. Even through the harshest summers and winters, they continue to grow strong and bear fruit.

Extra virgin olive oil is now probably the most extensively researched foodstuff on the planet, and its health benefits are evidence based. So – how can extra virgin olive oil contribute towards 'wellness?'

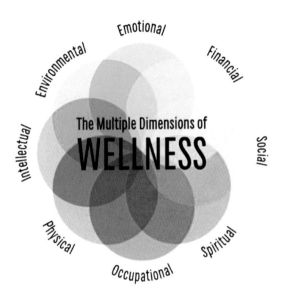

What Is Wellness?

Wellness is an active process of becoming aware of and making choices toward a healthy and fulfilling life. Wellness is more than being free from illness, it is a dynamic process of change and growth. Definitions include:

"...a state of complete physical, mental, and social well-being, and not merely the absence of disease or infirmity."

- *The World Health Organization*

"a conscious, self-directed and evolving process of achieving full potential."

- *The National Wellness Institute*

Maintaining an optimal level of wellness is crucial to living a higher quality of life. Wellness matters because every choice we make, everything we do, and every emotion we feel relates to our well-being. In turn, our well-being directly affects our actions and emotions. It's an ongoing circle.

There are reckoned to be eight dimensions of wellness: occupational, emotional, spiritual, environmental, financial, physical, social, and intellectual. Each dimension of wellness is interrelated with another. Each dimension is equally vital in the pursuit of optimum health.

How Extra Virgin Olive Oil Increases Emotional Wellness

Emotional wellness relates to understanding your feelings and coping effectively with stress. It is important to pay attention to self-care, relaxation, stress reduction, and the development of inner resources so you can learn and grow from experiences. The better you understand the processes and manage those feelings, the smoother the ride will be.

When incorporated into a varied healthy diet, including plenty of fruit, vegetables, and oily fish, extra virgin olive oil has been shown to contribute to decreasing the risk of depression.

According to a study from the University of Navarra and Las Palmas de Gran Canaria a diet rich in extra virgin olive oil can help to protect from mental illness.

The study included 12,059 volunteers and explored the dietary determinants of stroke, coronary disease, and other disorders. The research was conducted over a period of 6 years, during which time the researchers gathered data on lifestyle factors, including diet and medical history.

The results revealed that volunteers with a high intake of trans fats had up to 48 percent increased risk of depression compared to those who did not consumer those fats. In addition, the researchers also discovered that a higher intake of extra virgin olive oil and polyunsaturated fats was associated with a lower risk of depression.

This is one of a wealth of studies showing how extra virgin olive oil and the Mediterranean diet are associated with lower rates of depression.

Extra Virgin Olive Oil & The Environment

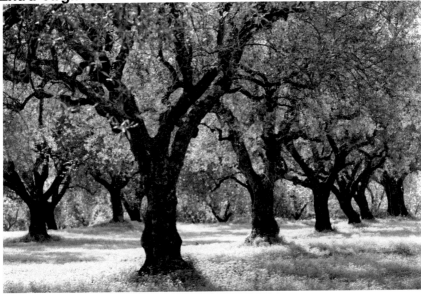

Environmental wellness inspires us to live a lifestyle that is respectful of our surroundings. This realm encourages us to live in harmony with the Earth by taking action to protect it. Environmental well-being promotes interaction with nature and your personal environment. Everyone can have a strong environmental conscious simply by raising their awareness.

A study by researchers from the University of Oxford and the University of Minnesota has demonstrated that foods that are considered to be healthy, such as whole-grain cereals, fruits, vegetables, legumes, nuts, and *olive oil*, also have the lowest environmental impact.

This extensive research by Michael A Clark, Marco Springmann, Jason Hill, and David Tilman, published in the journal Proceedings of the National Academy of Sciences (PNAS) (23) shows that eating healthier also means eating more sustainably and reveals a clear link between healthy food and environmental sustainability.

Food choices are shifting globally in ways that are negatively affecting both human health and the environment. Here the researchers considered how consuming an additional serving per day of each of 15 foods key food groups is associated with 5 health outcomes in adults and 5 aspects of agriculturally driven environmental degradation.

The researchers found that "while there is substantial variation in the health outcomes of different foods, foods associated with a larger reduction in disease risk for one health outcome are often associated with larger reductions in disease risk for other health outcomes. Likewise, foods with lower impacts on one metric of environmental harm tend to have lower impacts on others".

"Additionally, of the foods associated with improved health (whole grain cereals, fruits, vegetables, legumes, nuts, *olive oil*, and fish), all except fish have among the *lowest environmental impacts*, and fish has markedly lower impacts than red meats and processed meats. Foods associated with the largest negative environmental impacts—unprocessed and processed red meat—are consistently associated with the largest increases in disease risk.

Thus, dietary transitions toward greater consumption of healthier foods would generally improve environmental sustainability, although processed foods high in sugars harm health but can have relatively low environmental impacts. These findings could help consumers, policy makers, and food companies to better understand the multiple health and environmental implications of food choices".

As part of the study, the researchers examined the impact of consuming an additional serving per day of fifteen specific foods on five "health outcomes" in adults that are brought on by poor diets and account for nearly 40 percent of global mortality, specifically: mortality, type two diabetes, stroke, coronary heart disease, and colorectal cancer.

At the same time, the effects on five "aspects of agriculturally driven environmental degradation" were studied, including greenhouse gas emissions, land use, water use, acidification, and eutrophication (the last two are forms of nutrient pollution).

The foods included chicken, dairy, eggs, fish, fruits, legumes, nuts, *olive oil,* potatoes, processed red meat, refined grain cereals, sugar-sweetened beverages, unprocessed red meat, vegetables, and whole-grain cereals.

By comparing the five health and five environmental impacts of each food, the researchers determined that foods with the lowest environmental impacts often have the largest health benefits. Foods such as whole-grain cereals, fruits, vegetables, legumes, nuts, *olive oil*, and fish had the most positive impact on health while also having the lowest environmental impact (with the exception of fish).

Conversely, the foods with the largest environmental impacts, such as unprocessed and processed red meat, were also associated with the highest risk of disease. Minimally processed, health-boosting plant foods and olive oil were found to have a low environmental impact, but so did processed foods high in sugar that are harmful to health, such as sugar-sweetened beverages.

Reducing Financial Stress Through A Healthy Diet: Including Extra Virgin Olive Oil

Financial Wellness involves the process of learning how to successfully manage financial expenses. Money plays a critical role in our lives and not having enough of it impacts health as well as an academic or professional performance. Financial stress is repeatedly found to be a common source of anxiety and fear.

Extra virgin olive oil has been shown to have a significant impact on a range of chronic diseases. However, the cost of these diseases at both national and personal levels can be enormous. Cardiovascular diseases (CVDs) are the number 1 cause of death globally: more people die annually from CVDs than from any other cause.

An estimated 17.9 million people died from CVDs in 2016, representing 31% of all global deaths. Of these deaths, 85% are due to heart attack and stroke. In 2016, the cost of CVD in the USA alone was around $555Bn. This is expected to rise to $1.1Tr by 2035.

About 70 million adults in the US have hypertension – that's **1 in every 3**! and only around 52% of people with hypertension have it under control. It is also likely that many are walking around with the condition who don't even know they have it.

High blood pressure costs the USA around $48.6 billion each year. This total includes the cost of health care services, medications to treat high blood pressure, and loss of productivity from premature death.

1 in 3 Americans struggles with Crohn's disease, ulcerative colitis, irritable bowel syndrome (IBS), celiac disease, and other digestive conditions daily. Healthcare spending on a single patient with a digestive disease can range from $18k to $150k per year. Of this, specialty medications can cost up to $70k per person per year.

When we look at the high cost of specialty drugs used to treat advanced digestive disorders, it's easy to see how stigma and suffering in silence can eventually lead to a very expensive problem for both individuals and health services.

All of these chronic diseases and many more can be alleviated by regular consumption of high-quality extra virgin olive oil like Morocco Gold.

Intellectual Wellness: Extra Virgin Olive Oil Aids Cognitive Functions

Intellectual wellness is strengthened by continually engaging the mind. Doing so can help you build new skills and knowledge that inspire and challenge you and help you grow. You might choose different ways to keep your mind sharp, depending on your mood. For some, that's brain games and puzzles, or scholastic endeavours. Even simply engaging in intellectually stimulating conversations and debates can strengthen your intellectual wellness.

People who eat a Mediterranean-style diet, known to include fish, leafy vegetables, and extra virgin olive oil, increase their chances of better cognitive function, particularly later in life.

The scientific research by Edinburgh University, has shown that consuming lower amounts of red meat and following the principles of Mediterranean cuisine correlated with higher scores in memory and thinking tests in the over 70s.

Extra virgin olive oil is a key component of the Mediterranean diet, which is rich in fruits, vegetables, whole grains, and nuts.

These latest findings suggest that this primarily plant-based diet may have benefits for cognitive function as we get older.

Researchers involved in the study tested the thinking skills of more than 500 people aged 79 and without dementia. The participants completed tests of problem solving, thinking speed, memory, and word knowledge, as well as a questionnaire about their eating habits during the previous year.

More than 350 of the group also underwent a magnetic resonance imaging (MRI) brain scan to gain insights into their brain structure. The team used statistical models to look for associations between a person's diet and their thinking skills and brain health in later life.

The findings show that, in general, people who most closely adhered to a Mediterranean diet had the highest cognitive function scores, even when accounting for other factors, including childhood IQ, smoking, physical activity and health factors.

Occupational Wellness: How A Healthy Diet With Extra Virgin Olive Oil Can Help At Work

Occupational wellness is about enjoying your occupational endeavours and appreciating your contributions. This dimension of wellness encourages personal satisfaction and enrichment in one's life through work.

While many enlightened companies focus on physical activity in their corporate wellness program, they often don't prioritize the other pieces of the wellness puzzle – nutrition. According to the Institute for Health Metrics, poor nutrition has nearly three times the impact on health as low fitness. While more than two-thirds of the U.S. population classified as obese and 86 million Americans struggling with pre-diabetes, the need for better, more accessible nutrition education is evident.

Eating well in the workplace can have a significant impact on overall health and well-being. Nutritious foods can improve concentration and cognitive function, boosting an employee's workplace performance. It is well documented that employee well-being leads to higher creativity and productivity. The World Health Organization (WHO) has found that optimal nourishment can raise national productivity levels by 20%. Healthy employees are happier, calmer, more engaged, sleep better and get sick less often.

Providing healthy food options in the corporate setting is an effective way to get employees to stick to smart eating habits, which benefits both the individual and the company.

Social Wellness

Social relationships create support systems that can carry you through life's struggles. Harvard's Study of Adult Development ran for 80 years, collecting data on hundreds of participants. A recent study on a subset of this population, surviving octogenarians, investigated the connections between marital satisfaction, social lives, and happiness. Researchers found that participants who spent more time with others reported greater levels of happiness.

The impact of surrounding yourself with those that care for you can't be understated. When the demands of life increase and stress mounts, the ability to turn to someone for support and understanding is powerful. Building and maintaining these networks take time and energy, but the work is worth the effort. And it will continue to serve you throughout your life.

Spiritual Wellness

The spiritual pillar will look different for everyone because it's such a personal piece of overall wellness. It will play a stronger role in one person's life more than another, depending on how each person defines it.

Spirituality is commonly viewed as a sense of purpose, direction, or meaning, without which values can slip to the wayside, upending life's balance. Many cultivate their spirituality through meditation, prayer, or other activities that foster a connection to nature or a higher power.

Maintaining your spiritual wellness will look different for everyone. It's not about a specific religion or belief system. Spiritual health is about personalizing your journey. Some people might practice mindfulness as a way of checking in with their intentions, guiding their actions, and maintaining a values-based approach to life. How you choose to strengthen your spiritual health is up to you.

Extra Virgin Olive Oil And Physical Wellness

Physical wellness relates to maintaining a healthy body and seeking care when needed. Physical health is attained through exercise, eating well, getting enough sleep, and paying attention to the signs of illness, and getting help when needed.

Physical Wellness encourages us to care for our bodies through physical activity, proper nutrition, and a strong mind.

Being physically active is crucial to keeping your body in its top condition. A few proven benefits of physical activity are strengthened bones and muscles, reduced risk of disease and stroke, and more energy.

How A Diet With Extra Virgin Olive Aids Physical Wellness

Whether you are training for a competition or just building your fitness and strength for wellbeing and health, your results will be influenced by the diet you eat.

Choosing foods that are rich in healthy fats, such as extra virgin olive oil, can help improve your body's potential in many ways, including muscle recovery and increased energy levels.

For instance, this is particularly good news for runners who are considering following a Mediterranean diet to improve performance. According to a recent report in Runners World, the range of foods and good fats from nuts, seeds, and extra virgin olive oil can benefit runners in a number of ways.

By substituting heavily processed fats in meats and refined grains with more fruit, vegetables, and fish, runners can increase their carbohydrate intake, providing the quick-burning fuel that they need.

Nutrition

It is important to nurture your body by eating a well-balanced diet. Filling yourself with a variety of nutrients and vitamins will not only help prevent illness but will also keep your body functioning at its best.

This is where high quality extra virgin olive oil like Morocco Gold really helps. Research has demonstrated that regular use of high-quality extra virgin olive oil contributes towards:

Reducing of risk of cardiovascular diseases

Beneficial effects on ulcers and gastritis

Maintaining the digestive tract in good health.

Helping to reduce blood pressure

Helping to control healthy cholesterol levels

Easing or preventing diabetes

Lessening the severity of osteoporosis

If you think of your body as a highly tuned machine – extra virgin olive oil like Morocco Gold helps the machine run smoothly. It means that you are taking care of the 'inner self' and is one less thing to be concerned about in achieving overall wellness.

Understanding the relationship between your body's physical health and mental health is crucial in order to develop a balanced physical wellness. When you take the route to physical wellness, you will learn to understand how your body performs physically and be able to connect it to how you feel mentally. Physical wellness encourages principles of good health and knowledge, which affect behaviour patterns that lead to a healthy lifestyle. The following are a few suggestions to maintain an optimal level of physical wellness.

Engage in physical activity every day for 30 minutes.

Use stairs instead of the elevator or escalator and walk whenever possible.

Learn to recognize warning signs when your body begins feeling ill.

Eat a variety of healthy foods and control your meal portions.

Maintain a regular sleep schedule and get between 7-9 hours of sleep each night.

Practice safe sex.

This, in turn will help with…

Mental Well-Being

Having optimal levels of physical activity and maintaining proper nutrition are key to improving your overall intellectual and emotional wellness. Not only will you sharpen your thinking and learning abilities, but you will also enhance your sense of self-esteem and self-control.

CHAPTER 5.
THE HEALTH BENEFITS OF EXTRA VIRGIN OLIVE OIL

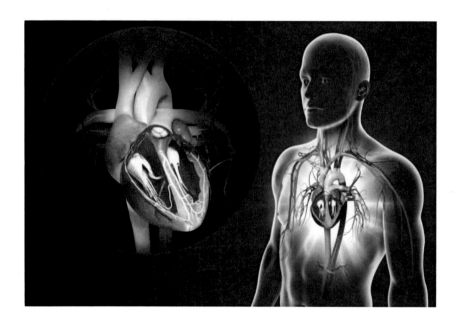

Reduced Risk Of Cardiovascular Diseases

Cardiovascular diseases (CVDs) are the number 1 cause of death globally: more people die annually from CVDs than from any other cause. (24)

An estimated 17.9 million people died from CVDs in 2016, representing 31% of all global deaths. Of these deaths, 85% are due to heart attack and stroke.

Most cardiovascular diseases can be prevented by addressing behavioural risk factors such as tobacco use, unhealthy diet and obesity, physical inactivity and harmful use of alcohol using population-wide strategies.

CVDs are a group of disorders of the heart and blood vessels. They include:

Coronary heart disease – a disease of the blood vessels supplying the heart muscle

Cerebrovascular disease – a disease of the blood vessels supplying the brain

Peripheral arterial disease – a disease of blood vessels supplying the arms and legs

Rheumatic heart disease – damage to the heart muscle and heart valves from rheumatic fever, caused by streptococcal bacteria

Congenital heart disease – malformations of heart structure existing at birth

Deep vein thrombosis and pulmonary embolism – blood clots in the leg veins, which can dislodge and move to the heart and lungs.

At the age of 24, your risk for CVD is just 20%. By age 45, your chances more than double to 50%. Over the age of 80, 90% of individuals have some form of CVD.

In 2016, the cost of CVD in the USA alone was around $555Bn. This is expected to rise to $1.1Tr by 2035. (25)

How Extra Virgin Olive Oil Helps Protect Against CVD

The increased focus on healthy food and healthy diet has seen more food lovers turn towards diets like the Mediterranean diet and the Keto diet. Whether this is for specific health reasons, a diet to lower cholesterol, a diet for high blood pressure, a diet for weight loss, or for overall wellness one of the key constituents that remains a constant is extra virgin olive oil, the original superfood.

What makes extra virgin olive oil so special is that it has stood the test of time as a superfood from the time of the ancients. Olive oil has long been considered sacred. The olive branch was often a symbol of abundance, glory, and peace. Over the years, the olive has also been used to symbolize wisdom, fertility, power, and purity.

In ancient Rome, olive oil was used for nearly everything in relation to their health. Roman medicine takes heavily from Greek doctors, who influenced European medicine for centuries, and Hippocrates, the father of modern medicine writes about over 60 different conditions or ailments that can be treated with olive oil.

Olive oil is now probably the most widely researched superfood on the planet and its many health benefits are evidence based and well understood. Thanks to the recent spotlight on the Mediterranean Diet, extensive research has been done on the phytonutrient composition of olive oil. What has been discovered is an extensive list of phytonutrients; one of the most praised is its polyphenols. The number of polyphenols found in Extra Virgin Olive Oil is truly amazing!

Polyphenols - Extra Virgin Olive Oils Powerful Antioxidant

Polyphenols are a potent antioxidant – one that can decommission a nasty molecule in your body called free radicals. Free radicals can ricochet around inside your body and harm good cells. Antioxidants, such as the polyphenols found in extra virgin olive oil, work to neutralize free radicals, protecting the body from their harmful effects. These antioxidants circulate in the body, hooking up with free radicals, unstable compounds thought to play a role in more than 60 different health conditions including cancer and atherosclerosis, as well as aging.

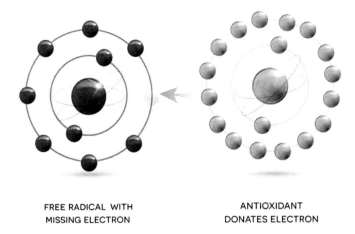

FREE RADICAL WITH
MISSING ELECTRON

ANTIOXIDANT
DONATES ELECTRON

Polyphenols, in other words, act as a powerful cell protector inside your body. Extra virgin olive oil like Morocco Gold is rich in polyphenols.

Several of the polyphenols found in olive oil, including hydroxytyrosol, oleuropein, and luteolin have shown to be especially helpful in avoiding unhealthy blood clotting by keeping our blood platelets in check.

Structures Of The Cardiovascular System

The cardiovascular system is responsible for transporting nutrients and removing gaseous waste from the body. This system is comprised of the heart and the circulatory system. Structures of the cardiovascular system include the heart, blood vessels, and blood. The lymphatic system is also closely associated with the cardiovascular system.

The Heart

The heart is the organ that supplies blood and oxygen to all parts of the body. This amazing muscle produces electrical impulses through a process called cardiac conduction. These impulses cause the heart to contract and then relax, producing what is known as a heartbeat. The beating of the heart drives the cardiac cycle, which pumps blood to cells and tissues of the body.

Blood Vessels

Blood vessels are intricate networks of hollow tubes that transport blood throughout the entire body. Blood travels from the heart via arteries to smaller arterioles, then to capillaries or sinusoids, to venules, to veins, and back to the heart. Through the process of microcirculation, substances such as oxygen, carbon dioxide, nutrients, and wastes are exchanged between the blood and the fluid that surrounds cells.

Blood

Blood delivers nutrients to cells and removes wastes that are produced during cellular processes, such as cellular respiration. Blood is composed of red blood cells, white blood cells, platelets, and plasma. Red blood cells contain enormous amounts of a protein called haemoglobin. This iron containing molecule binds oxygen as oxygen molecules enter blood vessels in the lungs and transport them to various parts of the body.

After depositing oxygen to tissue and cells, red blood cells pick up carbon dioxide (CO_2) for transportation to the lungs where CO_2 is expelled from the body.

Circulatory System

The circulatory system supplies the body's tissues with oxygen rich blood and important nutrients. In addition to removing gaseous waste (like CO_2), the circulatory system also transports blood to organs (such as the liver and kidneys) to remove harmful substances.

This system aids in cell to cell communication and homeostasis by transporting hormones and signal messages between the different cells and organ systems of the body. The circulatory system transports blood along with pulmonary and systemic circuits. The pulmonary circuit involves the path of circulation between the heart and the lungs. The systemic circuit involves the path of circulation between the heart and the rest of the body. The aorta distributes oxygen rich blood to the various regions of the body.

Lymphatic System

The lymphatic system is a component of the immune system and works closely with the cardiovascular system. The lymphatic system is a vascular network of tubules and ducts that collect, filter, and return lymph to blood circulation. Lymph is a clear fluid that comes from blood plasma, which exits blood vessels at capillary beds. This fluid becomes the interstitial fluid that bathes tissues and helps to deliver nutrients and oxygen to cells. In addition to returning lymph to circulation, lymphatic structures also filter the blood of microorganisms, such as bacteria and viruses. Lymphatic structures also remove cellular debris, cancerous cells, and waste from the blood. Once filtered, the blood is returned to the circulatory system.

Extra Virgin Olive Oil And The Cardiovascular System

Lowering your risk of cardiovascular problems is an area upon which several recent studies on Extra Virgin Olive Oil have focused. Chronic inflammation is a risk factor for many types of cardiovascular disease, and Extra Virgin Olive Oil has well-documented anti-inflammatory properties.

One place we don't want excessive ongoing inflammation is within our blood vessels. Our blood supply is just too important for maintaining the health of all our body systems, and it cannot effectively support our body systems when compromised with ongoing inflammation. Given this relationship, it's not surprising to see cardiovascular benefits of Extra Virgin Olive Oil rising to the top of the health benefits provided by this remarkable oil.

From a variety of different research perspectives, we know that daily intake of extra virgin olive oil in amounts as low as one tablespoon per day reduces inflammatory processes within our blood vessels. By reducing these processes, extra virgin olive oil also reduces our risk of inflammation-related cardiovascular diseases like atherosclerosis.

Yet anti-inflammatory benefits are not the only cardiovascular benefits provided by extra virgin olive oil. Two other broad types of heart-related benefits are well documented for this oil. The first type is lessened risk of forming unwanted blood clots. While blood clotting is a natural and healthy process required for the healing of wounds and prevention of excessive bleeding, clotting in the arteries can ultimately result in a heart attack or stroke.

One risk factor for unwanted clotting in our arteries is excessive clumping together of our platelet blood cells. This clumping process is also called "aggregation." Regular incorporation of extra virgin olive oil into a meal plan has been shown to lessen the risk of this excessive aggregation, and the reason that researchers refer to extra virgin olive oil as an "anti-aggregatory" oil.

The other broad area of cardiovascular benefits involves improved levels of circulating fats in our bloodstream, as well as protection of those fats from oxygen-related damage. Decreased levels of total cholesterol and LDL cholesterol following consumption of extra virgin olive oil are findings are the vast majority of studies that have analysed this relationship.

Yet equally important, the cholesterol molecules that remain in our blood also appear to be better protected from oxygen-related damage (oxidation). Since fats and cholesterol belong to a broader technical category called "lipids," damage to the fats and cholesterol in our bloodstream is typically referred to as "lipid peroxidation." And it is precisely this lipid peroxidation process that gets reduced through incorporation of extra virgin olive oil into a meal plan.

Cardiovascular Disease

Atherosclerosis is the build-up of fatty plaques on the walls of arteries. Fatty plaque known as atheroma (yellow) has built-up on the inner wall and is blocking about 60% of the artery width. Atherosclerosis leads to irregular blood flow and clot formation, which can block the coronary artery resulting in heart attack.

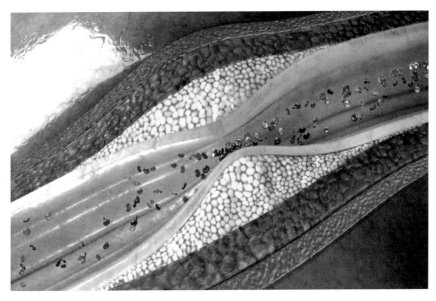

According to the World Health Organisation, cardiovascular disease is the leading cause of death for people world-wide. Cardiovascular disease involves disorders of the heart and blood vessels, such as coronary heart disease, cerebrovascular disease (stroke), elevated blood pressure (hypertension), and heart failure. These include:

Hypertension - persistently elevated blood pressure (high blood pressure) in the arteries. It is associated with the development of disorders such as atherosclerosis, heart attack, stroke, and can cause kidney damage.

Atherosclerosis - artery walls become hardened due to build-up of plaque (fatty deposits). It causes decreased blood supply to tissues and may lead to blood clots, stroke, aneurysm, or heart disease.

Aneurysm - a bulging in a weakened area of an artery that could rupture and cause internal bleeding.

Coronary artery disease (heart disease) - narrowing or blockage in the coronary arteries, which supply blood directly to the heart muscle. Complete blockage of blood flow will cause a heart attack.

Stroke - death of brain cells (neurons) due to lack of blood supply.

Heart failure - the heart is not able to supply enough blood to body tissues. It is caused by conditions such as hypertension, heart disease, and cardiomyopathy (chronic disease of the heart muscle).

It is crucial that the organs and tissues of the body receive proper blood supply. Lack of oxygen means death, therefore having a healthy cardiovascular system is vital for life. In most cases, cardiovascular disease can be prevented or greatly diminished through behavioural modifications. Individuals wishing to improve cardiovascular health should consume a healthy diet, exercise regularly, and abstain from smoking.

Imagine your body as a highly complex, high-performance engine. High quality extra virgin olive oil like Morocco Gold is nature's highest performance engine oil, to keep your body well-tuned and running smoothly over a lifetime.

Extra Virgin Olive Oil And The Digestive System

"All disease begins in the gut."

Hippocrates, father of modern medicine

People with digestive disease often suffer in silence because of the stigma associated with digestive symptoms. Many won't even discuss gut trouble with their doctors. When they finally do, it's because the pain, blood, fatigue, or constant bowel disruptions have become unbearable. Severe symptoms result in missed workdays, ER visits, emergency surgeries, and finally, long-term prescriptions.

Rising Cost Of Digestive Diseases

1 in 3 Americans struggles with Crohn's disease, ulcerative colitis, irritable bowel syndrome (IBS), celiac disease, and other digestive conditions daily. Healthcare spending on a single patient with a digestive disease can range from $18k to $150k per year. Of this, specialty medications can cost up to $70k per person per year. (26)

When we look at the high cost of specialty drugs used to treat advanced digestive disorders, it's easy to see how stigma and suffering in silence can eventually load to a very expensive problem for both individuals and health services.

Understanding Digestive Disorders

Digestive conditions can be brought on by stress, diet, and medications with little or no warning. Episodic flares lead to ER admissions and hospitalizations with very costly treatments. For people with digestive disease, following medication regimens can be very challenging, especially if they have other medical conditions to deal with. This can often result in poor outcomes, which, you guessed it, means even greater healthcare costs.

The digestive system provides fuel for the entire human body. It essentially supports all the body's other systems. When the digestive system is out of balance with an abnormal ratio of good to bad microbes, some unpleasant digestive conditions can creep up, causing chronic inflammation and a host of unpleasant symptoms. Diarrhoea, constipation, and pain are only part of it. Extreme fatigue, nausea, eye and mouth sores, skin conditions like eczema and psoriasis, and mental health disorders like depression and anxiety are all closely linked to digestive health.

Add to that poor diets, allergies, and busy lifestyles, and gut trouble is becoming a very big and very expensive problem.

How Does Extra Virgin Olive Oil Help?

We all have likely heard that extra virgin olive oil is one of the healthiest oil choices for cooking and eating. Extra virgin olive oil is high in fat, but most of it is heart-healthy monounsaturated fat, according to the American Heart Association. Choosing extra virgin olive oil over less healthy fats, such as butter, may benefit your heart and lower your cholesterol level. As if these benefits were not enough, extra virgin olive oil may also contribute to healthy digestion.

As soon as we consume extra virgin olive oil like Morocco Gold it has several effects all the way along with the digestive system. As far back as in ancient times it was recommended for assorted digestive disorders, and its beneficial properties are now being corroborated by epidemiological studies and a wealth of scientific data.

Once you swallow your food, your body takes over by secreting acids and other compounds that help break down the food and transport the nutrients it contains throughout your body. According to M. Carmen Ramirez-Tortosa and Parveen Yaqoob, authors of "Olive Oil and Health," extra virgin olive oil encourages the production of peptides, which support healthy digestion and aid in nutrient absorption. Regular consumption of extra virgin olive oil will keep your gut working efficiently by taking what it needs for good health and eliminating the rest in your waste.

Extra Virgin Olive Oil & The Stomach

Eating quickly, as well as eating high-fat foods, can cause gastric reflux or heartburn. Heartburn is characterized by a burning sensation in your stomach, throat, or oesophagus due to a high concentration of acid from your body attempting to digest these unhealthy types of food. A study published in the 2004 issue of Gracas y Aceites, a journal that focuses on the roles of fat and oils in the human diet, notes in that extra virgin olive oil may reduce the secretion of gastric acid.

Extra virgin olive oil reduces the risk of acid reflex and prevents gastric juices from traveling back up from the stomach to the oesophagus. Extra virgin olive oil inhibits gastric acid's motility. Because of this, the stomach's gastric content releases more gradually and slowly into the duodenum, making one feel fuller, having better digestion, and benefiting full nutrient absorption in the intestine.

Extra Virgin Olive Oil & The Hepatic-biliary System

One of the effects of extra virgin olive oil on the hepato-biliary system is that it is a cholagogue, ensuring optimal bile drainage and full emptying of the gall bladder. Another effect is that it is cholecystokinetic, i.e., it stimulates the contraction of the gall bladder, which is extremely helpful in the treatment and prevention of disorders of the bile ducts. It stimulates the synthesis of bile salts in the liver, and it increases the amount of cholesterol excreted by the liver.

In short, owing to its beneficial effect on the muscle tone and activity of the gall bladder, extra virgin olive oil stimulates the digestion of lipids because they are emulsified by the bile, and it prevents the onset of gallstones.

Extra Virgin Olive Oil & The Pancreas

Your pancreas is often an overlooked part of the digestive system, but it is essential for hormone production and for producing enzymes the small intestine needs to digest your food. Extra virgin olive oil is particularly beneficial to your pancreas because it only requires your pancreas to produce a small number of digestive enzymes, which means that it is working less, reports the before mentioned study in Gracas y Aceites. This benefits your pancreas by keeping it strong and healthy. The June 2000 issue of the Journal of Epidemiology and Community Health adds that extra virgin olive oil may also offer protection from pancreatic cancer.

When extra virgin olive oil is consumed, the pancreas releases a small amount of secretion, helping the organ efficiently and effectively carry out its purpose within the digestive system. Researchers recommend extra virgin olive oil to patients who have pancreatic problems, including cystic fibrosis, chronic pancreatitis, pancreatic failure, and malabsorption syndromes among others.

Extra Virgin Olive Oil & The Intestines

Your large and small intestines are essential for digesting your food and getting the nutrients throughout your body. Eating extra virgin olive oil in place of less healthy oils can improve the efficiency of your intestines. Extra virgin olive oil also encourages your intestines to absorb more of the vitamins and minerals from the foods you eat, which makes it beneficial for individuals suffering from digestive disorders, reports the 2004 study in Gracas y Aceites.

New research is also showing that polyphenols in extra virgin olive oil may help balance the bacteria in our digestive tract, slowing the growth of unwanted bacteria. On this list of polyphenols are: oleuropein, hydroxytyrosol, tyrosol and ligstroside. Some of these polyphenols are specifically able to inhibit the growth of the Helicobacter pylori bacterium; the bacterium that leads to stomach ulcers and other unwanted digestive problems. Yet another category of polyphenols called secoiridoids, continues to be a focus in research on prevention of digestive tract cancers.

Extra Virgin Olive Oil Can Boost Beneficial Gut Bacteria

Taking care of the microbes in our guts is one of the best ways to keep our digestive system working well and protect our immune system. That means packing as many fresh fruit and vegetables, whole grains, and Mediterranean staples like extra virgin olive oil into our cooking as we can.

Recent studies have shown that people who ate diets rich in plant-based foods and fish – akin to the famous Mediterranean diet – had higher collections of inflammation-fighting bacteria in their guts.

Extra Virgin Olive Oil Can Help Reduce Blood Pressure

About 70 million adults in the US have hypertension – that's **1 in every 3**! and only around 52% of people with hypertension have it under control. It is also likely that many are walking around with the condition who don't even know they have it. (27)

High blood pressure costs the USA around $131 billion each year. This total includes the cost of health care services, medications to treat high blood pressure, and loss of productivity from premature death. (27)

In 2014 Public Health England (PHE) revealed that diseases caused by high blood pressure are estimated to cost the NHS over £2 billion every year. Over 5 million people are unaware they have high blood pressure, yet it affects more than 1 in 4 adults and is one of the biggest risk factors for premature death and disability in England. (28)

High blood pressure can lead to diseases including heart disease, stroke, vascular dementia, and chronic kidney disease. High blood pressure, which can often be prevented or controlled through lifestyle changes, accounts for 12% of all visits to GPs in England.

The figures also showed that by reducing the blood pressure of the nation, £850 million of NHS and social care spending could be avoided over 10 years. If just 15% more people, unaware they have high blood pressure, are diagnosed, £120 million of NHS and social care spending could be avoided over 10 years. If another 15% more people, currently being treated for high blood pressure, controlled it better, a further £120 million of NHS and social care spending could be avoided over 10 years.

So, high blood pressure is a huge deal. High blood pressure is often characterized as a "silent killer" because it can cause permanent damage throughout the body without any obvious symptoms. Tragically, by the time the problem becomes obvious, it is sometimes too late to reverse the damage.

What Is Blood Pressure?

Blood pressure is a measure of the force that your heart uses to pump blood around your body. Blood pressure is measured in millimetres of mercury (mmHg) and is given as 2 figures: systolic pressure – the pressure when your heart pushes blood out; diastolic pressure – the pressure when your heart rests between beats. For example, if your blood pressure is "140 over 90" or 140/90mmHg, it means you have a systolic pressure of 140mmHg and a diastolic pressure of 90mmHg.

As a general guide, ideal blood pressure is considered to be between 90/60mmHg and 120/80mmHg. High blood pressure is considered to be 140/90mmHg or higher, low blood pressure is around 90/60mmHg or lower.

High blood pressure is often related to unhealthy lifestyle habits, such as smoking, drinking too much alcohol, being overweight, and not exercising enough. Left untreated, high blood pressure can increase your risk of developing several serious long-term health conditions, such as coronary heart disease and kidney disease.

Blood Pressure And Why It Matters

Blood travels from the heart via arteries to smaller arterioles, then to capillaries or sinusoids, to venules, to veins, and back to the heart. Blood pressure refers to the force pushing outward on the walls of your arteries. The more forcefully that the blood pumps, the more that the arteries are required to stretch to allow the blood to flow easily. Over time, if that force is too great, the tissue that makes up the arterial walls can become stressed and damaged.

This can lead a wide range of problems. For example, it makes arteries more vulnerable to infiltration and accumulation of cholesterol. It also can destabilize any existing arterial plaques, which increases the risk of them rupturing and inducing heart attacks.

Healthy blood pressure levels are an indicator of how clear the body's arteries are. When blood pressure levels get out of balance, they can signal a potential heart attack or stroke. High blood pressure levels are often caused by atherosclerosis, also called hardening of the arteries, which occurs when oxidized particles of LDL cholesterol stick to the walls of the arteries. Eventually, these particles build up and form plaque, narrowing the blood vessels and putting a heavier workload on the heart as it pumps oxygenated blood to the entire body.

How Does Extra Virgin Olive Oil Aid Blood Pressure?

Polyphenols have been shown to reduce morbidity and/or slow down the progression of cardiovascular, neurodegenerative, and cancer diseases. The mechanism of action of polyphenols strongly relates to their antioxidant activity. Polyphenols are known to decrease the level of reactive oxygen species in the human body. In addition, health-promoting properties of plant polyphenols comprise anti-inflammatory, anti-allergic, anti-atherogenic, anti-thrombotic, and anti-mutagenic effects. There is a body of research demonstrating their ability to modulate the human immune system by affecting the proliferation and activity of white blood cells, as well as the production of cytokines or other factors that participate in immunological defence.

Polyphenol Oleuropein

One of the specific polyphenols in Morocco, Gold extra virgin olive oil that directly combats the build-up of plaque within the arteries is called oleuropein. Oleuropein has been found by scientists to prevent the LDL cholesterol from oxidizing and sticking to the arterial walls.

Oleuropein is a natural phenolic compound found in olive leaves and green olives, including the olive's skin and flesh, from which olive oil is transferred. It causes the bitter taste in extra virgin olive oil.

Health Benefits Of Oleuropein

Oleuropein health benefits include antioxidant and natural anti-inflammatory activity, low blood glucose values, and free radicals removal. In addition, oleuropein has been linked to cardioprotective and neuroprotective activity.

Oleuropein belongs to a group of coumarin derivatives called secoiridoids. It was found to be effective against various strains of bacteria, viruses, fungi, and moulds, or even parasites. Oral treatment with oleuropein results in fewer blood vessels proving strong anti-angiogenic properties. Phenolic compounds (oleuropein, protocatechuic acid) in extra virgin olive oil have also been shown to inhibit macrophage-mediated LDL oxidation. Leaf and olive fruit extracts containing oleuropein protect insulin-producing β-cell line (INS-1) against the deleterious effect of cytokines.

Extra Virgin Olive oil And Hypertension: Clinical Trials

From a chronological perspective, one of the earliest randomized clinical studies assessing the antihypertensive effect of extra virgin olive oil dates to the late 1980s. Here, the antihypertensive effect of a high-fat diet enriched in extra virgin olive oil was compared to that of a reference diet, low in fat and rich in carbohydrate in a sample of 17 healthy subjects. After 36 days, systolic blood pressure (SBP) and diastolic (DBP) were significantly reduced in both experimental arms, with no significant difference between tested diets, thus suggesting, for the first time, a chance of regulating blood pressure (BP) by manipulating the amount of dietary extra virgin olive oil. Some years later, these results were confirmed in a group of 15 type-2 diabetic subjects, in which even more powerful antihypertensive effects by a diet enriched in extra virgin olive oil as compared with a high-carbohydrate diet were observed. (29)

Further Studies

Saturated fat diets are associated with the higher blood pressure, but there have been few good studies on whether the reverse is true; can unsaturated fats lower blood pressure, and are some unsaturated fats better than others?

A well-designed study published by researchers from the University of Naples, Italy fed 23 subjects a diet rich either in monounsaturated fatty acids (MUFA) such as are found in high quality extra virgin olive oil or polyunsaturated fatty acids (PUFA) such as are found in sunflower oil for one year.

At 26.6% of calories from fat, the experimental diet was also low in total fat. The study was double blinded, with neither subjects nor researchers aware of which oil was being used. Subjects were told to cook with given oil, and men were told to add 40g and women to add 30g of oil after cooking. The study participants experienced no change in weight during the year.

In their words, "the main result of our investigation was a straightforward reduction in antihypertensive tablet consumption when patients were given extra virgin olive oil, whereas drug consumption was only mildly affected by sunflower oil."

The need for common blood pressure drugs such as atenolol, HCTZ, and nifedipine was cut in half after just 4 months on the olive oil diet, whereas drug consumption was only mildly affected by sunflower oil. Cholesterol and triglyceride levels were also slightly lower while on the olive oil diet. There is as many as 5 mg of antioxidant polyphenols (absent in sunflower oil) in every 10 grams of olive oil. Antioxidants also reduce nitric acid levels, a substance in the body known to raise blood pressure.

Readers with concerns over high blood pressure should consult their doctor.

Extra Virgin Olive Oil Can Help Fight Inflammatory Diseases

Inflammation is a critical response to potential danger signals and damage to organs in our body. In diseases such as rheumatoid arthritis, lupus, ulcerative colitis, Crohn's disease, and others, the immune system turns against the bodies' organs. These painful and, in some cases, progressively debilitating conditions can take a toll on people's quality of life and create both societal and economic burdens.

The inflammatory process in the body serves an important function in the control and repair of injury. Commonly referred to as the inflammatory cascade, or simply inflammation, it can take two basic forms, acute and chronic. Acute inflammation, part of the immune response, is the body's immediate response to injury or assault due to physical trauma, infection, stress, or a combination of all three. Acute inflammation helps to prevent further injury and facilitates the healing and recovery process.

When inflammation becomes self-perpetuating, however, it can result in chronic or long-term inflammation. This is known as chronic inflammation and lasts beyond the actual injury, sometimes for months or even years. It can become a problem itself and require medical intervention to control or stop further inflammation-mediated damage.

Chronic inflammation can affect all parts of the body. Inflammation can also be a secondary component of many diseases. For example, in atherosclerosis, or hardening of the arteries where chronic inflammation of blood vessel walls can result in plaque build-up in the arteries, arterial or vascular blockages, and heart disease. Chronic inflammation also plays a significant role in other diseases and conditions, including chronic pain, poor sleep quality, obesity, physical impairment, and overall decreased quality of life.

The Cost Of Inflammatory Diseases

While it is difficult to measure the precise economic impact of chronic inflammation since this impact spans into almost all areas of chronic disease, as an example, in Europe the direct healthcare cost incurred by patients affected by Inflammatory Bowel Disease (IBD) has been estimated to be €4.6–5.6 billion per year.

In 2010, the cost of chronic obstructive pulmonary disease (COPD) in the U.S. was projected to be approximately $50 billion, which includes $30 billion in direct health care expenditures and $20 billion in indirect costs.

Economic burden to the U.K. NHS due to COPD was estimated at £982 million pounds in direct and indirect costs combined.14 The annual cost of treating COPD in Europe is estimated to be €38.6 billion. (30)

Types Of Inflammation

Inflammation is a process that protects the body from infection and foreign substances, such as bacteria and viruses. Inflammation helps the body by producing white blood cells and other substances. Sometimes, the immune system triggers an inflammatory response inappropriately. This is the case with autoimmune diseases. The body compensates by attacking its own healthy tissues, acting as if they are infected or abnormal.

When the inflammation process starts, chemicals in the white blood cells are released into the blood and the affected tissues to protect the body. The chemicals increase blood flow to the infected or injured body areas, causing redness and warmth in those locations. These chemicals may also cause leaking of fluids into tissues, resulting in swelling. This protective process will also stimulate nerves and tissues, causing pain.

Inflammation is classified as either acute or chronic. Acute inflammation is short-term, while chronic inflammation is long-lasting and even destructive.

Acute Inflammation

Acute inflammation may include the heat of a fever or warmth in the affected area. Acute inflammation is a healthy and necessary function that helps the body to attack bacteria and other foreign substances anywhere in the body. Once the body has healed, inflammation subsides.

Examples of conditions that cause acute inflammation include:

Acute bronchitis, which causes inflammation of the airways that carry air to the lungs.

An infected ingrown toenail.

A sore throat related to the flu.

Skin cuts and scratches.

Dermatitis, which describes multiple skin conditions including eczema, which causes red, itchy inflamed rashes in areas where the skin flexes (such as inside the elbows and behind the knees).

Sinusitis, which can cause short-term inflammation in the membranes of the nose and surrounding sinuses (usually the result of a viral infection) physical trauma.

Chronic Inflammation

Chronic inflammation, on the other hand, may continue to attack healthy areas if it doesn't turn off. It can occur anywhere in the body and may trigger any number of chronic diseases, depending on the area of the body affected.

Examples of conditions that cause chronic inflammation include:

Inflammatory arthritis, which covers a group of conditions distinguished by inflammation of joints and tissues (including rheumatoid arthritis, lupus, and psoriatic arthritis).

Asthma, which causes inflammation of the air passages that carry oxygen to the lungs. Inflammation causes these airways to become narrow and breathing to become difficult.

*Periodontiti*s, which causes inflammation of gums and other supporting teeth structures. It is caused by bacteria triggered by local inflammation.

Inflammatory bowel disease (IBD). IBD refers to Crohn's disease and ulcerative colitis. Both these conditions cause chronic inflammation in the gastrointestinal (GI) tract that eventually causes damage to the GI tract.

5 Cardinal Signs Of Inflammation: Pain, Heat, Redness, Swelling, And Loss Of Function

Interestingly, inflammation is a biological process that your body uses to help protect you. It is important to note, however, that not all five cardinal signs are present in every instance of inflammation. Moreover, the inflammatory process could be silent and not cause noticeable symptoms.

A cardinal sign is a major symptom that doctors utilize to make a diagnosis. In the case of inflammation, there are five cardinal signs that characterize the condition: pain, heat, redness, swelling, and loss of function.

Doctors and researchers sometimes refer to the five cardinal signs of inflammation by their Latin names:

Dolor (pain).

Calor (heat).

Rubor (redness).

Tumor (swelling).

Functio laesa (loss of function).

Pain

Inflammation can cause pain in joints and muscles. When inflammation is chronic, a person will experience high levels of pain sensitivity and stiffness. The inflamed areas may be sensitive to touch.

With both acute and chronic inflammation, pain is the result of inflammatory chemicals that stimulate nerve endings, causing the affected areas to feel more sensitive.

Heat

When inflamed areas of the body feel warm, it is because there is more blood flow in those areas. People with arthritic conditions may have inflamed joints that feel warm to the touch. The skin around those joints, however, may not have the same warmth. Whole-body inflammation may cause fevers because of the inflammatory response when someone has an illness or infection.

Redness

Inflamed areas of the body may appear red in colour. This is because blood vessels of inflamed areas are filled with more blood than usual.

Swelling

Swelling is common when a part of the body is inflamed. It is the result of fluid accumulating in tissues either throughout the body or in the specific affected area. Swelling can occur without inflammation, especially with injuries.

Loss of Function

Inflammation may cause loss of function, related to both injury and illness. For example, an inflamed joint cannot be moved properly, or it can make it difficult to breathe due to a respiratory infection.

Additional Signs and Complications

When inflammation is severe, it may cause additional signs and symptoms. This may include a general feeling of sickness and exhaustion. Inflammation due to illness may have dangerous complications, including a condition called sepsis. Sepsis occurs when the body's immune system overwhelmingly responds to a serious infection, which leads to generalized, life-threatening tissue damage.

Inflammation is a necessary part of the healing process and usually nothing to worry about. But when inflammation is chronic, it can be a serious health problem. Anyone experiencing ongoing inflammation should talk to their doctor about determining the source of inflammation and getting appropriate treatment to avoid any serious complications. (31)

Foods That Cause Inflammation

Foods that have been identified as causing inflammation and should be limited as much as possible include:

Refined carbohydrates, such as white bread and pastries

French fries and other fried foods

Soda and other sugar-sweetened beverages

Red meat (burgers, steaks) and processed meat (hot dogs, sausage)

Margarine, shortening, and lard

Not surprisingly, the same foods on an inflammation diet are generally considered bad for our health, including sodas and refined carbohydrates, as well as red meat and processed meats.

"Some of the foods that have been associated with an increased risk for chronic diseases such as type 2 diabetes and heart disease are also associated with excess inflammation," says Dr. Frank Hu, professor of nutrition and epidemiology in the Department of Nutrition at the Harvard School of Public Health. "It's not surprising since inflammation is an important underlying mechanism for the development of these diseases."

Unhealthy foods also contribute to weight gain, which is itself a risk factor for inflammation. Yet in several studies, even after researchers took obesity into account, the link between foods and inflammation remained, which suggests weight gain isn't the sole driver. "Some of the food components or ingredients may have independent effects on inflammation over and above the increased caloric intake," Dr. Hu says. (32)

A Healthy Diet Helps Combat Inflammation

One of the most powerful tools to combat inflammation comes not from the pharmacy but from the grocery store. "Many experimental studies have shown that components of foods or beverages may have anti-inflammatory effects," says Dr. Hu.

Choose the right anti-inflammatory foods, and you may be able to reduce your risk of illness. Consistently pick the wrong ones, and you could accelerate the inflammatory disease process.

Studies confirm that eating foods commonly part of the Mediterranean diet can do the following:

- Lower blood pressure
- Protect against chronic conditions, ranging from cancer to stroke

- Help arthritis by curbing inflammation
- Benefit your joints as well as your heart
- Lead to weight loss, which can lessen joint pain

Extra Virgin Olive Oil: Part Of An Anti-Inflammatory Diet

To reduce levels of inflammation, aim for an overall healthy diet. If you're looking for an eating plan that closely follows the tenets of anti-inflammatory eating, consider the Mediterranean diet, which is high in fruits, vegetables, nuts, whole grains, fish, and healthy oils like extra virgin olive oil.

In addition to lowering inflammation, a more natural, less processed diet can have noticeable effects on your physical and emotional health. "A healthy diet is beneficial not only for reducing the risk of chronic diseases but also for improving mood and overall quality of life," Dr. Hu says.

Anti-Inflammatory Benefits Of Extra Virgin Olive Oil

Phenols and polyphenols serve as the core substances that give extra virgin olive oil its unique anti-inflammatory properties. Researchers have determined that small amounts of extra virgin olive oil, as low as one tablespoon per day, can lower inflammatory signalling in our body, including levels of interleukin-6 (IL-6) and tumour necrosis factor alpha (TNF-alpha).

Interestingly, in Mediterranean-type diets that include daily intake of extra virgin olive oil, not only is there less production of signalling molecules like TNF-alpha, but there is also less activity by the cell receptors for these pro-inflammatory molecules. (This decreased receptor activity has been shown for tumour necrosis factor receptor 60 (TNFR 60) and tumour necrosis factor receptor 80 (TNFR 80). Levels of C-reactive protein (CRP) have also been showing to decrease with a daily intake of extra virgin olive oil.

In addition, scientists have shown that individuals who regularly consume extra virgin olive oil have reduced activity of their pro-inflammatory cyclo-oxygenase 1 (COX-1) and cyclo-oxygenase 2 (COX-2) enzymes, as well as reduced levels of related molecules including thromboxane B2 and leukotriene B4. Two molecules that are known to increase during inflammatory disease processes, vascular cell adhesion molecule-1 (VCAM-1) and intercellular adhesion molecule 1 (ICAM-1), have also been shown to decrease in amount following intake of extra virgin olive oil.

In this anti-inflammatory context, it is also worth noting that oxidative stress, a process that often parallels the process of chronic inflammation, is reduced by regular consumption of extra virgin olive oil. One common blood marker used to monitor oxidative stress is the formation of substances called F2-isoprostanes, and studies have shown 10-15% lower levels of this blood marker following extra virgin olive oil intake.

Importantly, the anti-inflammatory benefits of extra virgin olive oil do not depend on large levels of intake. In most studies, these benefits become statistically significant with as little as one tablespoon of extra virgin olive oil per day.

The anti-inflammatory benefits of extra virgin olive oil also appear to increase with daily intake above this level. An average daily extra virgin olive oil amount of 2 tablespoons per day is enough to provide strong anti-inflammatory benefits.

So which polyphenols in our extra virgin olive oil act as an anti-inflammatory?

The Anti-inflammatory Effect Of Polyphenol Oleuropein Aglycone (OA)

Oleuropein aglycone is a glycosylated Seco-iridoid, a type of bitter phenolic compound found in green olive skin, flesh, seeds, and leaves. The term oleuropein is derived from the botanical name of the olive tree, Olea Europaea. The chemical formula is: $C_{25}H_{32}O_{13}$.

Oleuropein aglycone is one of the chief polyphenols found in extra virgin olive oil. It is getting more and more global attention within the scientific and medical communities due to its biological properties, including in anti-Alzheimer's disease, anti-breast cancer, anti-inflammatory, anti-hyperglycemic effect, and anti-oxidative properties.

OA is derived from the de-glycosylation of oleuropein that exists in the leaves and stones of the olive fruit during the maturation period and is obtained during the pressing of the olives.

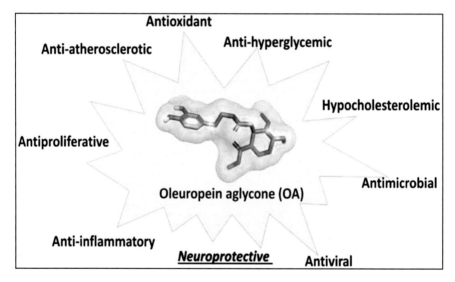

Inflammation is a complex immune response to pathogens, damaged cells, or irritants, and enables during infection or injury. Pain from inflammation is something most people experience at some point in their lives and a common daily occurrence for many people with arthritis OA plays an anti-inflammatory role during chronic inflammation and improves tissue damage associated with collagen-induced arthritis.

In addition, OA may be responsible for inhibiting cyclooxygenase (COX) enzymes. COX is an enzyme that forms prostanoids, prostaglandins, prostacyclins, and thromboxanes, which are all contributors to the inflammatory response. Therefore, OA can play an effective role in anti-inflammatory activities. (33)

Anti-inflammatory Polyphenol p-HPEA-EDA (Oleocanthal)

p-HPEA-EDA, otherwise known as Oleocanthal, belongs to the Tyrosol family of polyphenols. It is the dialdehydic form of decarboxymethyl ligstroside aglycone. It is synonymous with p-HPEA-Elenolic acid Di-Aldehyde and Ligstroside-aglycone di-aldehyde. Its chemical formula is $C_{17}H_{20}O_5$

The Oleocanthal molecule is responsible for the peppery / stinging sensation at the back of your throat when you ingest certain extra virgin olive oils. In fact, this is how the molecule got its name, 'oleo' means oil, and 'canth' is Greek for stinging or prickly.

The importance and uniqueness of Oleocanthal in extra virgin olive oil are that it has strong antioxidant and anti-inflammatory properties. Its anti-inflammatory action on the body is very similar to ibuprofen, one of the non-steroidal anti-inflammatory drugs most widely consumed.

Extra Virgin Olive Oil Helps Control Healthy Cholesterol

High cholesterol is when you have too much of a fatty substance called cholesterol in your blood. It is mainly caused by eating fatty food, not exercising enough, being overweight, smoking, and drinking alcohol. It can also run in families. You can lower your cholesterol by eating healthily and getting more exercise. Some people also need to take medicine. Too much cholesterol can block your blood vessels. It makes you more likely to have heart problems or a stroke. High cholesterol does not cause symptoms. You can only find out if you have it from a blood test.

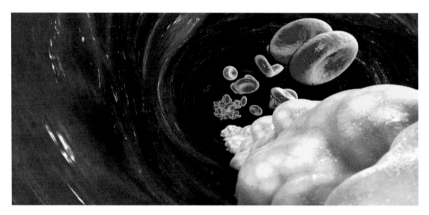

Cholesterol travels through the blood on proteins called "lipoproteins." Two types of lipoproteins carry cholesterol throughout the body:

LDL (low density lipoprotein) sometimes called "bad" cholesterol, makes up most of your body's cholesterol. High levels of LDL cholesterol raise your risk for heart disease and stroke.

HDL (high density lipoprotein) or "good" cholesterol absorbs cholesterol and carries it back to the liver. The liver then flushes it from the body. High levels of HDL cholesterol can lower your risk of heart disease and stroke.

High Cholesterol in the United States

In 2015–2016, more than 12% of adults age 20 and older had total cholesterol higher than 240 mg/dL

More than 18% had high-density lipoprotein (HDL, or "good") cholesterol levels less than 40 mg/dL.[1]

Slightly more than half of the U.S. adults (55%, or 43 million) who could benefit from cholesterol medicine are currently taking it.

93 million U.S. adults age 20 or older have total cholesterol levels higher than 200 mg/dL

Nearly 29 million adult Americans, have total cholesterol levels higher than 240 mg/dL

7% of U.S. children and adolescents ages 6 to 19 have high total cholesterol.

Having high blood cholesterol raises the risk for heart disease, the leading cause of death, and stroke, the fifth leading cause of death. (34)

A normal total cholesterol level for adults without heart disease is less than 200 mg/dL. An HDL cholesterol level of 60 mg/dL and above is considered protectivo against heart disease, while a level less than 50 mg/dL for women or 40 mg/dL for men is considered a major risk factor for heart disease

Lowering Cholesterol: Comparative Studies - Statins & The Mediterranean Diet

Nearly twenty years ago, two landmark randomized clinical trials appeared in The Lancet, which forever changed the course of medicine for patients with coronary heart disease (CHD). The 4S study employed a cholesterol-lowering statin drug and reported a 30% mortality reduction. The Lyon Diet

Heart Study utilized the Mediterranean diet and reported a 70% mortality reduction. (35)

Subsequent studies of the Mediterranean diet have confirmed these findings and have also shown a reduced risk of cancer, diabetes, and Alzheimer's disease. Subsequent statin studies have led the United States Food and Drug Administration to issue warnings regarding the increased risk of diabetes and decreased cognition with statin drugs. Paradoxically, statins have gone on to become a multi-billion-dollar industry and the foundation of many cardiovascular disease prevention guidelines, while the Mediterranean diet has often been ignored.

The authors of the study, Robert Dubroff and Michel de Lorgeril concluded, "we believe this statin-centric cholesterol-lowering approach to preventing CHD may be misguided". They further found.

The dramatic benefits of the Mediterranean diet are likely due to multiple mechanisms which do not directly involve cholesterol. Independent of cholesterol metabolism is the true fatal complications of coronary atherosclerosis - thrombotic coronary occlusion, acute myocardial ischemia, left ventricular dysfunction, and malignant arrhythmias.

The haemostatic system appears to be a principal modulator of atherosclerotic plaque formation and progression, and the Mediterranean diet can favourably alter elements of the coagulation cascade. Plaque rupture and intra-plaque haemorrhage lead to progressive atherosclerosis, thrombosis causes acute coronary syndromes, and sudden cardiac death is the main cause of cardiac mortality.

At the genetic level large scale, genome-wide association studies have identified 46 loci directly linked to CHD, yet most of these loci have no apparent relation to cholesterol or traditional risk factors. Although we can't change our genes, epigenetic studies have shown that the Mediterranean diet can favourably alter the expression of atherogenic genes, whereas a recent cholesterol-lowering statin trial failed to demonstrate a similar effect. (36)

The Health Benefits Of Extra Virgin Olive Oil: A Further Study

Montserrat Fitó, Ph.D., is the senior author of research by the Cardiovascular Risk and Nutrition Research Group at the Hospital del Mar Medical Research Institute in Barcelona, Spain. Fitó and the team's findings were published in the American Heart Association's journal Circulation. (37)

There are two types of molecules called lipoproteins that carry cholesterol in the blood: low-density lipoprotein (LDL) and high-density lipoprotein (HDL).

LDL is known as "bad" cholesterol, since having high levels of LDL can bring about plaque build-up in the arteries, which can result in heart disease and stroke. HDL is known as "good" cholesterol; HDL (good) absorbs cholesterol and carries it to the liver where it is flushed from the body. Having high levels of HDL (good) reduces heart disease and stroke.

The research team aimed to determine whether eating a Mediterranean diet enriched with extra virgin olive oil or nuts over a long period of time would improve the beneficial properties of HDL (good) cholesterol in humans.

Fitó and collaborators randomly selected a total of 296 individuals who had a high risk of heart disease and were participating in the Prevención con Dieta Mediterránea study. The participants had an average age of 66 and were assigned to one of three diets for a year.

The first diet was a traditional Mediterranean diet enriched with around 4 tablespoons of extra virgin olive oil per day. The second a traditional Mediterranean diet supplemented with a fistful of nuts each day. The third diet was a healthful "control" diet that contained a reduced amount of red meat, high-fat dairy products, processed foods, and sweets.

Both Mediterranean diets emphasized the inclusion of fruit, vegetables, legumes (such as beans, chickpeas, lentils, and whole grains), and moderate amounts of fish and poultry.

Blood tests were conducted at the start and end of the study to measure LDL (bad) and HDL (good) levels.

Extra Virgin Olive Oil-enriched Mediterranean Diet Enhanced HDL function

The researchers found that total and LDL (bad) cholesterol levels were only reduced in the healthful control diet. While none of the three diets significantly increased HDL (good) levels, the two Mediterranean diets improved HDL (good) function, and the improvement was more pronounced in the group enriched with extra virgin olive oil.

The Mediterranean diet enriched with extra virgin olive oil improved HDL (good) functions, such as reversing cholesterol transport, providing antioxidant protection, and enabling vasodilation.

Reverse cholesterol transport is the process in which HDL (good) removes cholesterol from plaque in the arteries and takes it to the liver. Antioxidant protection is the ability of HDL (good) to counteract the oxidation of LDL (bad). Oxidation of LDL (bad) triggers the development of plaque in the arteries.

Lastly, vasodilator capacity, which relaxes the blood vessels, keeps them open, and keeps the blood flowing, is improved by the Mediterranean diet with extra virgin olive oil.

Although the control diet was rich in fruits and vegetables like the two Mediterranean diets, the diet was shown to have an adverse impact on HDL's (good) anti-inflammatory properties. This negative impact was not observed in the Mediterranean diets. A reduction in HDL's (good) anti-inflammatory capacity is linked with a greater risk of heart disease.

"Following a Mediterranean diet rich in virgin olive oil could protect our cardiovascular health in several ways, including making our 'good cholesterol' work in a more complete way."

Montserrat Fitó (38)

Conclusion

The debate over the cholesterol hypothesis and statins has raged for decades. Some may point to the recent decline in cardiovascular deaths in the United States as proof of statin effectiveness, but this view fails to incorporate the impact of smoking cessation, lifestyle changes, and dramatic improvements in heart attack survival rates due to timely reperfusion and the availability of external and implantable defibrillators. Others may argue that statins are started too late in life to be effective (the horse may already be out of the barn) and reference Mendelian randomization studies, which show that rare individuals with genetically low cholesterol levels have a much lower incidence of CHD.

However, this concept should not be extrapolated to the 99.99% of us who lack these genes and fails to explain how the Mediterranean diet reduces mortality within months of initiation. In 1996 Nobel laureates Brown and Goldstein anticipated the eradication of coronary disease in their *Science* editorial, "Exploitation of recent breakthroughs - proof of the cholesterol hypothesis, discovery of effective drugs, and better definition of genetic susceptibility factors - may well end coronary disease as a major public health problem early in the next century". (39)

History has proven otherwise, and the global prevalence of CHD, despite worldwide statin usage and cholesterol lowering campaigns, has reached pandemic proportions. Coronary heart disease is an extremely complex malady, and the expectation that it could be prevented or eliminated by simply reducing cholesterol appears unfounded. After twenty years, we should concede the anomalies of the cholesterol hypothesis and refocus our efforts on the proven benefits of a healthy lifestyle incorporating a Mediterranean diet to prevent CHD. (40)

Note: Readers with concerns over Cholesterol levels should consult their doctor

Extra Virgin Olive Oil Eases Or Helps Prevent Diabetes

The American Diabetes Association (ADA) released new research on March 22, 2018, estimating the total costs of diagnosed diabetes rose to $327 billion in 2017 from $245 billion in 2012, when the cost was last examined. This figure represents a 26% increase over a five-year period.

The study, *Economic Costs of Diabetes in the U.S. in 2017*, was commissioned by the ADA and addressed the increased financial burden, health resources used, and lost productivity associated with diabetes in 2017.

People with diagnosed diabetes incur average medical expenditures of $16,752 per year, of which about $9,601 is attributed to diabetes. On average, people with diagnosed diabetes have medical expenditures approximately 2.3 times higher than what expenditures would be in the absence of diabetes.

For the cost categories analysed, care for people with diagnosed diabetes accounts for one in four health care dollars in the U.S., and more than half of that expenditure is directly attributable to diabetes. (41)

In the UK, the costs to the National Health Service (NHS) for treating diabetes took prominence in the media in November 2018 as the NHS bill for blood glucose-lowering drugs for the first time surpassed £1 billion.

Almost one in 20 general practitioners' (GP) prescriptions are now for diabetes treatment; the largest increase was for type 2 diabetes treatment. (42)

What Is Blood Sugar (Glucose)?

Blood sugar (glucose) is the key to keeping the working of the body in good condition. When blood sugar levels start to fluctuate, the body starts showing signs of unhealthy functioning.

Glucose plus healthy fat (monosaturated fats such as are found in extra virgin olive oil) is the preferred source of energy in the body. While glucose is important, it is also important to keep it in moderation. When we eat, our body immediately starts processing glucose. Enzymes breakdown with the help of the pancreas.

In some people (diabetics) they cannot completely rely on the pancreas to work. Diabetes is a condition where the pancreas doesn't produce adequate insulin.

Maintaining glucose levels is important for the normal functioning of the body. The ideal range of sugar levels is 90-130 mg/dL while fasting, whereas post meals, it needs to be less than 180 mg/DL.

Reasons Why Blood Sugar Rises:

Heavy meals

Stress

Underlying illness

Sedentary lifestyle

Skipping medication

Blood Sugar Levels And Extra Virgin Olive Oil

Regulation of blood sugar (glucose) especially after eating is one regulatory system that has a definite friend in extra virgin olive oil. One recent study on individuals diagnosed with impaired fasting glucose (IFG) helps explain the ability of extra virgin olive oil to improve blood sugar regulation. (43)

Like this name implies, IFG is a condition in which blood sugar levels are too high, even when no food is being eaten and digested. However, in this study, participants were given a little less than one tablespoon of extra virgin olive oil along with a familiar lunch meal of pasta, salad, fruit, and a slice of ham. When the participants' insulin and blood sugar levels were measured at one hour and two hours after lunch, their blood sugar levels were found to be significantly lower due to this added extra virgin olive oil.

Researchers for this study went one step further, however. They looked at potential ways in which extra virgin olive oil might have produced these desirable effects. What they found were higher levels of incretins, specifically glucagon-like peptide-1 (GLP-1) and glucose-dependent insulinotropic polypeptide (GIP) in the blood of participants after consuming extra virgin olive oil since these incretins are molecules that stimulate more insulin production, raising their levels resulted in more insulin secretion and more removal of sugars from the blood.

In short, these study participants achieved better insulin secretion and better regulation of blood sugar levels following their lunch meal through the addition of extra virgin olive oil.

How Can Extra Virgin Olive Oil Help Improve Blood Sugar Levels

Tyrosol is a key polyphenol in Morocco Gold extra virgin olive oil. Tyrosol is a phenylethanoid, a derivative of phenethyl alcohol. It is a natural phenolic antioxidant present in a variety of natural sources. The principal source for human diet is in high quality extra virgin olive oil like Morocco Gold. As an antioxidant, tyrosol can protect cells against injury due to oxidation.

Along with hydroxytyrosol, tyrosol is one of the most abundant polyphenols in extra virgin olive oil, where they occur as such or in the form of esters of elenolic acid. There is an increasing level of research into these polyphenols and their properties to determine which is the most significant contributor towards the range of health benefits associated with high quality extra virgin olive oil.

Its beneficial properties for human health are strongly related to the ability of the molecule to scavenge free radicals and reactive oxygen/nitrogen species as well as to activate endogenous antioxidant systems in the body. Free radical scavenging properties have been convincingly confirmed in studies on rats with alloxan-induced diabetes mellitus.

Extra Virgin Olive Oil & Diabetes: A Further Study

In a further study, conducted at Sapienza University in Roman, (44) researchers examined the health benefits of a traditional Mediterranean diet, including extra virgin olive oil for people with diabetes

This was a small study involving only 25 participants, all of whom ate a typical Mediterranean lunch consisting primarily of fruits, vegetables, grains, and fish on two separate occasions. For the first meal, they added 10g of extra virgin olive oil. For the second, they added 10g of corn oil. After each meal, the participant's blood glucose levels were tested. The rise in blood sugar levels was much smaller after the meal with extra virgin olive oil than after the meal with corn oil.

Lowering blood glucose and cholesterol may be useful to reduce the negative effects of glucose and cholesterol on the cardiovascular system," said Francesco Violo, lead author of the study.

The findings were consistent with previous studies, which have linked extra virgin olive oil to higher levels of insulin, making it beneficial to people with type 2 diabetes. More surprising, however, were the reduced levels of low-density lipoprotein (LDL), or "bad" cholesterol, associated with the extra virgin olive oil meal.

The researchers stressed that consuming extra virgin olive oil on its own is not going to provide the benefits observed during the study. Rather, it has to be consumed within the context of a balanced diet. (45)

Further Ways To Lower Blood Sugar

You should have foods you enjoy but keep a check on what goes inside the body because food can help in diabetes care and diabetes management. As well as extra virgin olive oil certain lifestyle choices that help manage blood glucose levels include;

Raw cooked food: Opt for low carb vegetables such as eggplants, tomatoes, sprouts, and mushrooms. You can top it with some pepper or garlic seasoning.

Green leafy food: If you enjoy salads, then you can try a spinach salad. They are rich in health and low in carb. You could top it with some chia seeds for the extra crunch.

Low calorie drinks: Water is best, but you do need an alternative sometimes. You could try some cinnamon tea. They are low carb and keep you feeling full.

Nuts & Seeds: Nuts prevent heart disease and control blood sugar levels. Nuts like almonds help regulate blood sugar. Seeds like flax seeds help improve fasting glucose levels and lower bad cholesterol.

Exercise: A sedentary lifestyle is the major cause of diabetes. It is essential that you invest in some low duty exercise daily along with your medication.

Individuals who are suffering from diabetes and related issues usually show drastic improvement in their development when they self-participate in diabetes management. It is recommended to track your blood glucose levels regularly using a glucometer to a keep track of your blood glucose level patterns. (46)

Extra Virgin Olive Oil Lessens The Severity Of Osteoporosis

One of the most common health problems in the United States, osteoporosis affects more than 44 million Americans and contributes to an estimated 2 million fractures each year. Fifty percent of women and 25% of men over the age of 50 will sustain fractures thanks to osteoporosis. Many fractures happen because of a fall, but even simple household tasks can cause severely osteoporotic bones to fracture. (51)

Skeletal mass and microarchitecture degenerate with aging, thus predisposing the elderly to skeletal fragility and fractures. The global estimate of osteoporotic hip fracture incidence in 2000 was nine million and resulted in more disability adjusted life years lost compared to common cancers excluding lung cancers. The prevalence of osteoporosis is predicted to rise exponentially with the accelerated expansion of elderly population, especially in developing countries. The tremendous economic and healthcare burdens caused by osteoporotic fractures deserve much attention from the medical and scientific community.

What Causes Osteoporosis?

Though the exact causes of osteoporosis are unknown, doctors have identified major factors that can lead to the disease.

Aging

Losing bone with age is a natural phenomenon and after the age of 35 the body builds less new bone to replace the loss of old bone. As a rule, your bone mass goes down as your age goes up, and thus your risk for osteoporosis increases.

Heredity

A family history of the disease, fair skin, and Caucasian or Asian descent can increase the risk for osteoporosis. This fact may help explain why some develop the disease early in life.

Nutrition And Lifestyle

A calcium-deficient diet, excessively low weight, and a sedentary lifestyle have all been linked to osteoporosis, along with smoking and excessive alcohol consumption.

Medications and Other Illness

Some medications, including steroids, and other diseases like thyroid problems have been linked to osteoporosis.

Treatment

Lost bone cannot be replaced, and as such, treatment focuses on preventing the condition from becoming worse. Treatment plans often involve work from physicians, orthopaedists, a gynaecologist, and an endocrinologist. In addition to including regular intake of extra virgin olive oil, exercise, and nutrition as part of your lifestyle choices, other treatments include:

Estrogen Replacement Therapy

Often offered to women at high risk for osteoporosis, estrogen replacement therapy (ERT) helps prevent bone loss and reduce fracture risk. The hormones also help prevent heart disease and improve cognitive function but can increase the risk for breast cancer.

Selective Estrogen Receptor Modulators

Known as SERMs, these anti-estrogens can increase bone mass, reduce fracture risk, and lower the risk for breast cancer.

Calcitonin

This medication is available in nasal spray form and helps increase bone mass and relieve pain.

Bisphosphonates

These significantly increase bone mass and help prevent spine and hip fractures.

How Does Extra Virgin Olive Oil Help To Keep Bones Healthy?

Adherence to a Mediterranean diet with extra virgin olive oil at its heart was associated with decreased fracture incidence in the European Prospective Investigation into Cancer and Nutrition Study (52), involving 188,795 subjects followed for nine years. The Mediterranean diet, including extra virgin olive oil was also associated with increased calcium absorption and retention and a decrease in urinary calcium excretion in male adolescents.

Olives and extra virgin olive oil are important components in the Mediterranean diet. A Mediterranean diet enriched with olive oil has been associated with increased levels of bone formation markers than non-enriched diet in elderly men.

Mice fed with olive oil also had higher apparent calcium absorption and calcium balance, but a lower serum calcium, phosphate, and magnesium level compared to groups fed with other lipids. It is thought that this could be attributed to the high phenolic content of extra virgin olive oil. These phenolic compounds, which include tyrosol, hydroxytyrosol, and oleuropein, exert prominent antioxidant and anti-inflammatory effects; thus, are potential candidate agents for osteoporosis prevention.

Extra Virgin Olive Oil & Bone Fractures: A Study

One recent study compared the number of bone fractures in a group of 870 study participants over a period of seven years to see if intake of extra virgin olive oil was associated with the number of reported bone fractures. When the study results were analysed, the researchers divided this large group into three categories.

In terms of their extra virgin olive oil intake, the lowest third of the study participants averaged 38 grams of extra virgin olive oil per day, approximately 3 tablespoons. The middle third averaged nearly 4 tablespoons (48 grams), and the top third averaged about 4.5 tablespoons (57 grams).

Participants in the highest category of extra virgin olive oil intake reported 51% fewer fractures than participants in the lowest category of extra virgin olive oil intake.

While all these extra virgin olive oil intake levels are fairly high, they nevertheless show a link between reduced risk of bone fracture and incorporation of extra virgin olive oil into an ordinary meal plan. It's also worth noting that numerous animal studies have shown increased bone formation in rats and mice that were given extra virgin olive oil in their feeding plan. This increased bone formation has also been specifically tied to the presence of two phenols, tyrosol and hydroxytyrosol in extra virgin olive oil.

Conclusion

Olives, extra virgin olive oil, or olive polyphenols have the potential to be developed as bone protective agents. This is supported by evidence derived from preclinical studies using animal models of osteoporosis and a limited number of human studies. The bone protective effects of olive and its products are attributed to their ability to increase bone formation and inhibit bone resorption by suppressing oxidative stress and inflammation. However, the exact pathways are still elusive and await future validation. Well-planned randomized controlled trials on olive and its derivatives are warranted to justify its use in osteoporosis prevention. (53, 54)

Anyone experiencing or at risk of the effects of osteoporosis should talk to their doctor to determine the appropriate course of treatment.

Extra Virgin Olive Oil Can Help Combat Osteoarthritis

Osteoarthritis (OA) is a form of arthritis that features the breakdown and eventual loss of the cartilage of one or more joints. Cartilage is a protein substance that serves as a "cushion" between the bones of the joints. Among the over 100 different types of arthritis conditions, osteoarthritis is the most common joint disease.

OA occurs more frequently as we age. Before age 45, osteoarthritis occurs more frequently in males. After 55 years of age, it occurs more frequently in females. In the United States, all races appear equally affected. Hand osteoarthritis, hip osteoarthritis, and knee osteoarthritis are much more common in seniors than younger people. A higher incidence of osteoarthritis exists in the Japanese population, while South-African blacks, East Indians, and Southern Chinese have lower rates. (55)

Osteoarthritis commonly affects the hands, feet, spine, and large weight-bearing joints, such as the hips and knees.

Osteoarthritis usually has no known cause and is referred to as primary osteoarthritis. When the cause of the osteoarthritis is known, the condition is referred to as secondary OA.

What Causes Primary Osteoarthritis?

As part of normal life, your joints are exposed to a constant low level of damage. In most cases, your body repairs the damage itself, and you do not experience any symptoms. But in osteoarthritis, the protective cartilage on the ends of your bones breaks down, causing pain, swelling, and problems moving the joint. Bony growths can develop, and the area can become red and swollen.

The exact cause is not known, but several things are thought to increase your risk of developing osteoarthritis, including:

Natural Ageing

Your risk of developing the condition increases as you get older. Primary (idiopathic) osteoarthritis, OA not resulting from injury or disease, is partly a result of natural aging of the joint. With aging, the water content of the cartilage increases, and the protein makeup of cartilage degenerates as a function of biologic processes. Eventually, cartilage begins to degenerate by flaking or forming tiny crevasses. In advanced osteoarthritis, there is a total loss of the cartilage cushion between the bones of the joints.

Joint Injury

Repetitive use of the worn joints and overusing your joint after an injury or operation when it has not had enough time to heal can mechanically irritate and inflame the cartilage, causing joint pain and swelling.

Loss Of Cartilage

Loss of the cartilage cushion causes friction between the bones, leading to pain and limitation of joint mobility. Inflammation of the cartilage can also stimulate new bone outgrowths (spurs, also referred to as osteophytes) to form around the joints.

Family History

Osteoarthritis occasionally can develop in multiple members of the same family, implying a hereditary (genetic) basis for this condition. Osteoarthritis is therefore felt to be a result of a combination of each of the above factors that ultimately lead to a narrowing of the cartilage in the affected joint.

Secondary Osteoarthritis

Secondary osteoarthritis is a form of osteoarthritis that is caused by another disease or condition. Conditions that can lead to secondary osteoarthritis include:

Obesity

Being obese puts excess strain on your joints, particularly those that bear most of your weight, such as your knees and hips. Obesity causes osteoarthritic by increasing the mechanical stress on the joint and therefore, on the cartilage. In fact, next to aging, obesity is the most significant risk factor for osteoarthritis of the knees.

Repeated Trauma Or Surgery To The Joint Structures

The early development of osteoarthritis of the knees among weightlifters is believed to be in part due to their high body weight. Repeated trauma to joint tissues (ligaments, bones, and cartilage) is believed to lead to early osteoarthritis of the knees in soccer players and army military personnel.

Interestingly, health studies have not found an increased risk of osteoarthritis in long-distance runners.

Abnormal Joints At Birth (Congenital Abnormalities)

Some people are born with abnormally formed joints (congenital abnormalities) that are vulnerable to mechanical wear, causing early degeneration and loss of joint cartilage. Osteoarthritis of the hip joints is commonly related to structural abnormalities of these joints that had been present since birth.

Gout

Crystal deposits in the cartilage can cause cartilage degeneration and osteoarthritis. Uric acid crystals cause arthritis in gout, while calcium pyrophosphate crystals cause arthritis in pseudogout.

Diabetes

Disorders such as diabetes, hemochromatosis, growth hormone disorders, are also associated with early cartilage wear and secondary osteoarthritis.

Symptoms Of Osteoarthritis

The main symptoms of osteoarthritis are joint pain and stiffness and problems moving the joint. Some people also have symptoms such as: - swelling - tenderness - grating or crackling sound when moving the affected joints

The severity of osteoarthritis symptoms can vary greatly from person to person and between different affected joints.

For some people, the symptoms can be mild and may come and go. Other people can experience more continuous and severe problems, which make it difficult to carry out everyday activities.

Almost any joint can be affected by osteoarthritis, but the condition most often causes problems in the knees, hips, and small joints of the hands.

You should see your GP if you have persistent symptoms of osteoarthritis so they can confirm the diagnosis and prescribe any necessary treatment.

Polyphenol Ligstroside-Aglycone (LA): It's Role In Combating Osteoarthritis

This polyphenol is synonymous with p-HPEA-Elenolic acid. It is a member of the Tyrosol family of polyphenols and has the chemical formula: $C_{19}H_{22}O_7$

While information on LA bioactivity is limited, a few years ago, LA was demonstrated to behave as an antioxidant. Furthermore, LA has been shown to have anti-inflammatory effects by controlling and downregulating NF-κB (NF-kB is a type of DNA that is thought to play a pivotal role in the initiation of osteoarthritis and the perpetuation of chronic inflammation in rheumatoid arthritis) as well as the potential to induce a caloric restriction-like state that affects the muscle, brain, fat tissue and kidney, particularly through activation and increased levels of sirtuins. (Sirtuins are a family of proteins that regulate cellular health. They play a key role in regulating cellular homeostasis, keeping cells in balance).

A Study Of Ligstroside-Aglycone In Treatment Of Osteoarthritis

In a recent study at the Faculty Of Pharmacy Seville and the Biomedical Research Institute Coruna (M.S. Meiss, M. Sanchez-Hidalgo, A. Gonzales-Benjumea) the effectiveness of LA on osteoarthritis (OA) was examined. (56)

Osteoarthritis is currently the most frequent cause of pain, deformity, and dysfunction in the elderly. It is a late-onset, complex disease of the joints, characterised by progressive failure of the extracellular cartilage matrix (ECM), together with changes in the synovium and subchondral bone.

OA persists as the most common form of arthritis worldwide and the sixth leading cause of disability. Unlike most tissues, articular cartilage does not contain blood vessels, nerves, or lymphatics, rather, articular cartilage is composed of a dense ECM with a sparse distribution of highly specialised cells called chondrocytes. Aberrant expression of degradative proteases or catabolic mediators is induced in OA chondrocytes that contributes to cartilage destruction.

To date, there is no definitive cure for this debilitating disease. The mechanism of disease progression in OA remains largely unknown, and thus, to date, a more personalised approach is required to aid patient disease management. Current treatments are targeted at reducing symptoms of the inflammatory reaction that occurs following the destruction of the essential joint cartilage. These treatments, however, do not prevent the significant pain associated with OA or the often-reported restriction of mobility and activity.

To address this unmet need, alternative approaches, including the use of polyphenols as a novel therapeutic intervention, are under examination. The objective of this study was to analyse if the polyphenols found in extra virgin olive oil can reverse the catabolic activity that contributes to cartilage destruction in OA.

Two polyphenols from extra virgin olive oil, oleocanthal (OLC), and ligstroside aglycone (LA), plus a chemically modified acetylated ligstroside aglycone (A-LA), and two marine polyunsaturated fatty acids, eicosapentaenoic acid (EPA) and docosahexaenoic acid (DHA), were examined as potential anti-inflammatory agents for OA.

The Results

Acetylated ligstroside showed the most promising results for implementation in treating OA as it reduced the expression of pro-inflammatory genes such as inducible nitric oxide (*iNOS*), matrix metalloprotease-13 (*MMP13*) and interleukin-1β (*IL1B*) at both RNA and protein levels; decreased nitric oxide (NO) levels from cartilage explants and reduced proteoglycan (PG) losses in human osteoarthritic cartilage explants and chondrocytes.

These results substantiate the role of polyphenols in OA with implications for therapeutic intervention and our understanding of OA pathophysiology.

Recently, data from the Osteoarthritis Initiative (OAI) have demonstrated that adherence to the Mediterranean diet is associated not only with better quality of life but also, significantly, with a lower prevalence of OA. Given that the general population can be viewed as at risk in the development of OA in later life, an approach that relies on dietary modification is attractive in terms of risk/benefit and, potentially, an approach that is more likely to be implementable. Indeed, as an alternative to traditional treatments, alternative modalities have come to the fore, including the effects of polyphenols as non-invasive treatments, based on the evidence that epigenetic changes aro triggered by dietary nutrients and contribute to the prevention of several diseases. (57)

Preventing osteoarthritis

It's not possible to prevent osteoarthritis altogether. However, you may be able to minimise your risk of developing the condition by avoiding injury and living a healthy lifestyle.

Exercise

Avoid exercise that puts strain on your joints and forces them to bear an excessive load, such as running and weight training. Instead, try exercises such as swimming and cycling, where the strain on your joints is more controlled.

Try to do at least 150 minutes of moderate aerobic activity (such as cycling or fast walking) every week, plus strength exercises on 2 or more days each week that work for the major muscle groups, to keep yourself generally healthy.

Posture

It can also help to always maintain good posture and avoid staying in the same position for too long. If you work at a desk, make sure your chair is at the correct height, and take regular breaks to move around.

Losing Weight

Being overweight or obese increases the strain on your joints and your risk of developing osteoarthritis. If you're overweight, losing weight may help lower your chances of developing the condition.

Finally, when arthritis symptoms persist, it is best to seek the advice of a health care professional who can properly guide the optimal management for each individual patient. Many other prescription medications are available for the treatment of osteoarthritis for patients with chronic, annoying symptoms.

Polyphenols In Extra Virgin Olive Oil have Anti-bacterial Properties

A recent study by researchers at the National Research Council's Institute of Food Sciences and the University of Salerno has shown that polyphenols from three different olive oil varieties have an inhibitory effect against several bacterial strains.

The tests were performed using 2.5 and 4.9 micrograms of the three polyphenol extracts against different pathogens. The results showed that the minimum concentration necessary to inhibit the growth of the pathogenic tester strains was low for all the polyphenolic extracts. This confirmed their general capacity to inhibit the growth of pathogenic or unwanted microorganisms.

All three extracts were effective in inhibiting the growth of Escherichia coli, a bacterium that is one of the causes of urinary tract infections. The three extracts also were found to be capable of inhibiting the growth of Pseudomonas Aeruginosa, a well-known pathogen that is responsible for the formation of biofilms.

Biofilms are densely packed communities of microbial cells that grow on living or inert surfaces and surround themselves with secreted polymers. Because the protective shell can keep out potential treatments, biofilms are at their most dangerous when they invade human cells or form on sutures and catheters used in surgeries. In American hospitals alone, thousands of deaths are attributed to biofilm-related surgical site infections and urinary tract infections.

"They gave us remarkable results in terms of their activity against pathogenic species, namely those that are responsible for the formation of biofilms. This could be a basis of complementary studies to formulate ideal drugs of natural origin, composed of optimal mixtures of polyphenols, which are able to exercise with the minimum effort, in terms of quantity, and the maximum result, namely against the greatest number of pathogens, their antibacterial efficacy," - Filomena Nazzaro, senior scientist at the National Research Council's Institute of Food Sciences, Italy (58)

Polyphenols In Extra Virgin Olive Oil Help Combat Cancer

Research studies are providing better and better documentation for the anti-cancer benefits of extra virgin olive oil. Early studies in this area were largely limited to research using rats and mice or research on cell cultures in the lab. But more recent studies have looked at people incorporating extra virgin olive oil into their everyday meal plan and have found encouraging results.

As few as 1–2 tablespoons of extra virgin olive oil per day have been associated with decreased risk of breast, respiratory tract, and digestive tract cancers. In the case of the digestive tract, reduced risk seems more likely in the upper tract (stomach and small intestine) than in the lower digestive tract (large intestine, including the colon).

Scientists have looked at several different mechanisms that might allow extra virgin olive oil to provide these anti-cancer effects. One group of studies have focused on the secoiridoids, oleuropein, and decarboxylmethyl oleuropein, and determined that these extra virgin olive oil phytonutrients help shift some of our metabolic pathways in the direction of better stress resistance. In addition, the overall phenolic content of extra virgin olive oil has been associated with a decreased ability of cancer cells to regenerate. At least some of this effect involves the ability of two phenols in extra virgin olive oil—tyrosol and hydroxytyrosol—to block activity of an enzyme called matrix metalloproteinase 2 (MM-2).

The multiplication of cancer cells depends on an adequate supply of oxygen, and to obtain this supply of oxygen, cancer cell growth is often accompanied by the formation of new blood vessels (through a process called angiogenesis). Because the activity of MM-2 is needed to trigger this process of new blood vessel formation, substances that block MM-2 activity can also lessen the likelihood of new blood vessel formation. The tyrosol and hydroxytyrosol in Extra Virgin Olive Oil may decrease the likelihood of cancer cell regeneration by interfering with angiogenesis and lowering the supply of oxygen that would otherwise be available for new blood vessel formation.

Investigating Polyphenolic Compounds In Extra Virgin Olive Oil

Many studies have identified the components of extra virgin olive oil which confer health benefits, but few have tested the effect of high phenolic extra virgin olive oil on cancer.

Dr Limor Goren, Hunter College of the City University of New York, and Dr David Foster, (59) has recently carried out research to explore the anti-cancer effects of oleocanthal, a phenolic compound found in extra virgin olive oil. Oleocanthal is the molecule thought to be responsible for the 'peppery' sensation at the back of your throat when you take certain extra virgin olive oils. In fact, this is how the molecule got its name, 'oleo' means oil, and 'canth' is Greek for stinging or prickly.

The study has shown that oleocanthal specifically kills human cancer cells, but not normal, non-cancerous cells. The authors suggest that this is due to the ability of oleocanthal to induce the death of cancer cells through lysosomal membrane permeabilisation (LMP). Permeabilising the lysosomal membrane allows digestive enzymes stored inside this organelle to be released, which preferentially causes cell death in cancer cells. In their latest study, they found that oleocanthal was able to induce LMP in cancer cells grown in the laboratory. The team tested whether the observed damage to lysozymoc was due to permcation of the membrane, or whether something else could have damaged them. Interestingly, purified lysosomes outside the cell were not affected by oleocanthal, indicating that oleocanthal only induces lysosomal permeability in a cellular context.

One limitation identified by Dr Goren is that this work used purified oleocanthal, therefore it is not known whether oleocanthal in a more natural form, i.e., as a component of olive oil, can cause a similar outcome. To overcome this, the group carried out a similar experiment using olive oil enriched cell culture media and found similar results.

Furthermore, recognising that different olive oils have different oleocanthal concentrations due to their origin, harvest time, and processing methods, the researchers tested a variety of olive oils to determine their respective concentrations of oleocanthal, which ranged from very low to very high. The olive oils that had high oleocanthal content completely killed cancer cells in vitro (in a petri dish), in a manner similar to purified oleocanthal. The olive oils with average oleocanthal content reduced viability, but to a lesser extent. Those with no oleocanthal had no effect on cell viability.

Oleocanthal Extends Life Span Of Mice With Tumours

In addition to the findings in cancer cells discussed above, Dr Goren and colleagues also found that injection of oleocanthal into mice engineered to develop pancreatic neuroendocrine tumours, reduced their tumour burden and extended the lifespan of the mice. More specifically, the oleocanthal injections extended the lives of the mice by an average of four weeks. Based on lifespan conversion, if oleocanthal has the same effect in humans, it might extend human life by more than 10 years.

Oleocanthal Induces LMP And Cathepsin Leakage In Cancer Cells

A separate study, which was conducted by scientists from Weill Cornell Medicine, Rutgers University, and Albert Einstein College of Medicine (60), in addition to Hunter College, supports the findings of how oleocanthal kills cancer cells. As mentioned previously, oleocanthal induces damage to cancer cells' lysosomes, cell components that contain enzymes used to break down larger molecules like proteins. The oleocanthal degrades the integrity of the lysosomal membrane, releasing the enzymes into the cells' cytoplasm, which leads to cell death. Cancer cells often have larger and more numerous lysosomes, making them more vulnerable to oleocanthal than other cells.

Furthermore, many cancer cells upregulate the formation and turnover of lysosomes and their enzymatic contents.

Extra virgin olive oil is a tried and tested natural remedy for many ailments, but in order to potentially harness its benefits for a cancer treatment, more needs to be understood about the type of olive oil and the dose required in humans. In addition, this study shows that it is not just any olive oil that is important, but the high concentration of phenolic compounds of the selected oil that is crucial.

Extra Virgin Olive Oil And Breast Cancer

In a study carried out by Dr Javier Menendez and colleagues from the Catalan Institute of Oncology in Spain (61) to investigate the effects of extra virgin olive on breast cancer cells grown in laboratory cultures, it was shown that the substances in extra virgin olive oil work in a similar way to the drug Herceptin by reducing the concentration of HER2 protein that helps HER2-positive breast cancer to grow.

Using a method called solid-phase extraction, researchers extracted the polyphenols from commercially available extra virgin olive oil. These were then added to the growth medium for HER2-positive and HER2-negative breast cancers to see what effect they had on the tumour cells.

They found that the polyphenols from the extra virgin olive oil reduced the levels of HER2 protein and also increased tumour cell death. HER2 is a protein found on the surface of some cancer cells, including breast cancer. This protein can bind to another molecule (known as the human epidermal growth factor), which then encourages the growth and division of the tumour cells. Not all breast cancers have the HER2 protein on their surface; it is estimated that one in five women with breast cancer will have HER2 receptors.

Several laboratory tests were then carried out to determine how fast the tumour cells were growing, their metabolic activity, whether the phenol caused cell death, whether the phenol had an effect on levels of HER2 protein and whether or not HER2 protein was activated in the presence of the phenol. The results from these tests were compared with those from tests performed on breast cancer cells that were not cultured with the phenols.

The Study Findings

This study found that phenols extracted from extra virgin olive oil have an effect on HER2-positive breast cancer cells grown in culture in the laboratory. The researchers found that some single phenolic compounds (including hydroxytyrosol, tyrosol, and others) and all the polyphenols (several phenols joined together) from extra virgin olive oil induced "strong tumoricidal effects" in breast cancer cells that had HER2 protein on their surface. The phenols also reduced the levels of HER2 protein and its activation.

The Conclusions

The researchers concluded that the phenols in extra virgin olive oil can cause degradation of the HER2 protein on breast cancer cells. This may mean they can be used as a basis for the design of new HER2-targeting agents.

Studies Show The Positive Effects Of Extra Virgin Olive Oil On Your Immune Response

Over the last year, the role of our immune system has been front of mind for most people, but did you know that extra virgin olive oil is one of the best foods for boosting your body's immune response?

Infections or infectious diseases are caused by viruses, bacteria, parasites, fungi, and various other disease-causing agents. Once an infection is contracted, the human body relies on the immune system to fight the infection through a range of cellular, inflammatory, and immune reactions. Although there are medications to treat infection, naturally derived food sources such as extra virgin olive oil also show promise in preventing and treating infection also.

Early in vitro studies showed that several polyphenols in extra virgin olive oil have antibacterial properties against human pathogens, particularly oleuropein, tyrosol, and hydroxytyrosol. In a 5-minute room temperature test, hydroxytyrosol, and tyrosol decreased the activity of Listeria monocytogenes, the bacteria contracted from contaminated food that causes the bacterial infection known as Listeriosis.

Decarboxymethyl elenolic acid (EDA), p-HPEA-EDA, and 3,4-DHPEA-EDA have been shown to have greater antimicrobial activity than the commercial disinfectants glutaraldehyde and ortho-phthalaldehyde. The phenolic compound oleocanthal has been shown to inhibit the growth of Helicobacter pylori bacteria, a bacteria associated with peptic ulcer and gastric cancer development.

Hydroxytyrosol and oleuropein have been shown to have antiviral activity in a dose-dependent manner. They were shown to inhibit the main viral fusing protein in human immunodeficiency virus (HIV)-1 target cells. Hydroxytyrosol has been shown to disrupt the influenza virus. Oleuropein has been shown to have anti-hepatitis B activity.

In recent times, researchers have begun to understand the role of intestinal microorganisms (gut microbes) in the overall health of the immune system. Therefore, protection against the growth of certain microorganisms can help in the treatment of some infectious diseases.

A study published in Journal of Nutritional Biochemistry, 2016, (62) established that changes in gut microbes in subjects with metabolic syndrome had immune-enhancing effects. The authors conclude that "the consumption of a Mediterranean diet, including extra virgin olive oil, increased the abundance of the Bacteroides genus member B. thetaiotaomicron and F. prausnitzii, which suggest that the consumption of this diet may increase or maintain a microbiota with anti-inflammatory capability."

Fatty acids, also known as dietary lipids, are also involved in the modulation of the immune system and inflammatory processes. Oleuropein aglycone inhibits the proinflammatory molecule TNF-a. Hydroxytyrosol has been shown to reduce TNF-a, and interleukin-1 beta with promising effects on other key pro-inflammatory molecules. Tyrosol has been shown to inhibit COX-2. And oleocanthal has extensive research surrounding its anti-inflammatory benefits for preventing and treating various health conditions.

A further study in Nutrition & Metabolism 2015, (63) aimed to determine the effect on immune responses when replacing oils in a typical American diet with extra virgin olive oil for a 3-month period. Forty-one obese or overweight subjects were randomized to extra virgin olive oil or a mixture of corn, soybean oil, and butter (CON). The extra virgin olive oil group saw decreases in blood pressure, increases in HDL cholesterol levels, and in direct relation to the immune system, increased anti-CD3/anti-CD28 stimulated T cell proliferation, showing clear immunological health benefits.

Overall, the results of both in vitro and in vivo studies show that extra virgin olive oil is beneficial for various infections and infectious diseases. Best of all, it's a natural food source that is readily available to everyone and comes with no side effects.

8 Steps to Help Support a Healthy Immune System

With all this science to get to grips with, it's worth remembering that sticking to just a few basic guidelines can help you fight off disease and infection. (64)

Eat A Balanced Diet

Include whole fruits, vegetables, lean proteins, whole grains, and plenty of water. A Mediterranean Diet is one option that includes these types of foods.

Don't smoke (or stop smoking if you do).

Drink alcohol in moderation

Perform moderate regular exercise.

Aim for 7-9 hours of sleep nightly.

Try to keep a sleep schedule, waking up and going to bed around the same time each day. Our body clock, or circadian rhythm, regulates feelings of sleepiness and wakefulness, so having a consistent sleep schedule maintains a balanced circadian rhythm so that we can enter deeper, more restful sleep.

Aim to manage stress

This is easier said than done but try to find some healthy strategies that work well for you and your lifestyle—whether that be exercise, meditation, a particular hobby, or talking to a trusted friend. Another tip is to practice regular, conscious breathing throughout the day and when feelings of stress arise. It doesn't have to belong—even a few breaths can help.

Wash hands throughout the day

When coming in from outdoors, before and after preparing and eating food, after using the toilet, after coughing or blowing your nose.

CHAPTER 6.
OLIVE OIL AND A HEALTHY LIFESTYLE

What Is A Healthy Lifestyle?

A healthy lifestyle is one that helps to keep and improve your health and well-being. There are many different things that you can do to live a healthy lifestyle, such as eating healthy, being physically active, maintaining a healthy weight, and managing your stress. However, a healthy lifestyle isn't just about healthy eating and exercise, it is also about taking care of the "whole you" – your physical, mental, emotional, and spiritual well-being. And that means taking care of you from the inside out.

How To Live A Healthy Lifestyle

Even though there are many common ways to live a healthy lifestyle, actually doing it looks different for everyone and means something different from one person to the next. Regardless of what you choose to do, living a healthy lifestyle is a key component to disease prevention, wellness, and longevity.

Being mindful of your diet, physical activity, and stress levels allows you to effectively balance all aspects of your life and the "whole you".

Eat More Fruit & Vegetables

Fruits contain lots of vitamins and minerals. As much as possible, you should consume your vitamins and minerals via your daily diet. Satisfy your palate with these nutritious fruits: Watermelon, Apricots, Avocado, Apple, Cantaloupe, Grapefruit, Kiwi, Guava, Papaya, Strawberries.

Like fruits, vegetables are important for good health. Experts suggest 5-9 servings of fruits/vegetables a day, but unfortunately, it may be difficult at times. However, when you can, include foods like kidney beans, black beans, asparagus, long beans, green beans, and carrots. Think about your favourite vegetables and how you can include more of them in your diet every day.

Cut Down On Processed Food

Processed foods are not good because most nutritional value is lost in the making of these foods and the added preservatives are bad for our health. Many processed foods contain a high amount of salt content, which leads to higher blood pressure and heart disease. Processed foods are anything that is not in its raw form. In general, most foods in supermarkets are processed — the more ingredients it has on the label (especially the ones ending with 'ite' or 'ate'), the more processed they are. Watch out for those with salt/sugar in the first 5 ingredients and go for unprocessed food as much as possible.

Drink More Water

Most of us don't drink enough water every day. With over 60% of our body made up of water, it is essential for our body to function. Water is needed to carry out body functions, remove waste, and carry nutrients and oxygen around our bodies. Since we lose water every day through urine, bowel movements, perspiration, and breathing, we need to replenish our water intake. Since food intake contributes about 20% of our fluid intake, that means we need to drink about 8-10 glasses a day to stay hydrated.

One way to tell if you're hydrated — your urine should be colourless or slightly yellow. If it's not, you're not getting enough water! Other signs include Dry lips, dry mouth, and little urination.

Exercise Regularly

If you can exercise, don't just a few times a week, but every day. Movement is key to a healthy life. Exercising daily can improve your health in many ways. It can help increase your life span, lower your risk of diseases, help you develop higher bone density, and lose weight.

One simple thing you can do is, especially for close distances, choose walking over riding, driving, or taking transportation. You can climb the stairs instead of taking the elevator. You can pick exercises that are easy to do at home or outside that you enjoy. When you enjoy the physical activities you choose for yourself, most likely you'll enjoy them and naturally want to do them. Exercise is about being healthy and having fun at the same time. Also, mixing up your exercises will keep them interesting.

«Νοῦς ὑγιής ἐν σώματι ὑγιεῖ». That's the ancient Greek saying which means "a healthy mind in a healthy body" and underlines the necessity for keeping both your mind and body in shape. Greece has a great tradition in sports -considering they were the ones who introduced The Olympic Games, as well as in extra virgin olive oil.

In mythology, the god Poseidon and the goddess Athena were competing for the same city. It was up to the people to decide, so each god offered a gift to the city. Poseidon created a water fountain, but the water was salty like the sea, so it wasn't much use. Athena, on the other hand, gave them an olive tree, which was better since it provided food, oil, and wood. She was the one chosen to be the protector of the city and this is how Athens took its name. Since then, the olive tree signified peace, wisdom, and victory and olive oil became a major part of their culture.

This is why the winners of the first Olympic Games, held in 776 BC, were crowned with branches of the sacred olive trees. And so were the winners of the Great Panathinea, a sports event held in Athens in honour of the goddess Athena.

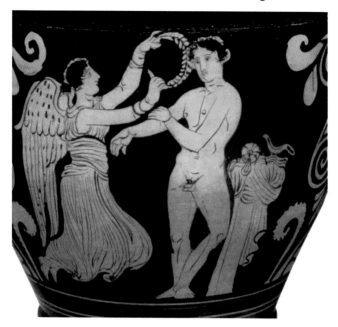

The winners of the Panathinea were also gifted with largely decorated amphoras filled with extra virgin olive oil. This olive oil was produced from specific olive trees growing on the famous rock of the Acropolis. Those trees were considered sacred, and the value of the olive oil, being symbolic and pecuniary was extremely high, as no one else, but the winners could possess it. Even nowadays, Marathon winners in the Olympic Games are crowned with olive branches, continuing a tradition of 3000 years.

However, the olive trees and oil did not have only symbolic and pecuniary significance. The ancient athletes also applied olive oil on their skin before a competition to protect their muscles, and they regularly consumed pure extra virgin olive oil.

Today, extra virgin olive oil remains as beneficial to today's athlete as ever and the Mediterranean diet, rich in fruits, vegetables, fish, and extra virgin olive oil as the only source of fat, is the ideal food model. In fact, good nutrition is an integral part of training which improves the mental well-being and ensures a better performance.

Energy Boost

To start with, the consumption of olive oil provides energy and fats essential to athletes. Fats may be saturated, polyunsaturated, monounsaturated, and trans-fat. It is wildly known that unsaturated fats are the best choice for athletes. Olive oil helps lower cholesterol levels and contributes to heart health and building bones. It is made up of mostly monounsaturated fatty acids in the form of oleic acid, a few saturated fats, and some polyunsaturated fats such as linoleic acid.

At its most basic, olive oil provides energy, something athletes never want to be without. Compared to the sedentary who should consume no more than 15% of their calories from fat, athletes need anywhere from 20%-30%. This is true for both endurance and high-intensity sports. Fat is the body's main fuel during low-intensity lengthy endeavours like triathlons and marathons, but it's just as necessary for high-intensity sports too. Carbohydrates may be the central fuel for high-intensity activities, but without fat, carbohydrate energy cannot be released.

Muscle Recovery

Muscles have a hard time during athletic training and need immediate recovery, which includes repair, strengthening, and muscle building. Olive oil is better than other fat sources in helping cells absorb cholesterol and convert it to testosterone, which is critical to the body's muscle building process. Moreover, its combination of oleic acids and polyunsaturated fatty acids work together to build bone tissue and allow the body to regenerate.

Breathe Deeply On Purpose

Oxygen is a vital source of life. You may know how to breathe, but are you breathing properly? Most of us don't breathe properly — we take only shallow breaths and breathe to 1/3 of our lung capacity. A full breath is one where your lungs are completely filled, your abdomen expands, and there's minimum movement in your shoulders.

There are many benefits of deep breathing, which include a reduction in stress and blood pressure, strengthening of abdominal and intestinal muscles, and relief of general body aches and pains. Deep breathing also helps with better blood flow, releasing toxins from the body, and aids in getting a better night's sleep.

Get Enough Sleep

Lack of sleep may lead to a host of health problems including obesity, diabetes, and even heart disease. Continued lack of sleep can affect your immune system and make you less able to fend off colds and the flu. So, it's important go get a good night's sleep.

You can do things to help you sleep better at night. You can avoid stimulants such as caffeine and nicotine close to bedtime. Also, while alcohol is well-known to help you fall asleep faster, too much close to bedtime can disrupt sleep in the second half of the night as the body begins to process the alcohol.

Exercise can also help you sleep better at night. As little as 10 minutes of aerobic exercise, such as walking or cycling, can drastically improve night-time sleep quality but please avoid strenuous workouts close to bedtime.

Reduce Your Stress Levels

To optimize physical wellness, it is critical to pay attention to the mind. From migraines to heart attacks, drugs and surgery may treat the immediate condition but do not address the underlying causes. There is almost always a stress connection.

There are more than 1,400 biochemical responses to stress, including a rise in blood pressure and accelerated heart rate. Those areas of the brain that trigger stress responses are fed by stress, causing even more stress creating a cycle of stress.

Stress changes the brain. It shrinks the part that helps us focus and perform and increases the part that sets off fear and anxiety. Stress feeds on itself, and chronic stress accelerates aging. We're more resilient when we're young, but over time, the hormones that help us beat stress are depleted.

Not worrying about your stress helps relieve it, but if you are not a naturally calm person, you can learn techniques to help manage your reaction to it. If you cannot change the events in your life that are causing stress, the goal is to change your response to it, so that the endorphins that calm the brain are released.

Stop Smoking And / Or Avoid Passive Smoking

Smoking can severely increase your risk of lung cancer, kidney cancer, esophageal cancer, heart attack, and more. Smoking "light" cigarettes do not decrease health risks either. If you do smoke, stop now and do it not only for yourself but also your family and friends.

Second-hand smoking (breathing in air from smokers) can cause many of the same long-term diseases as direct smoking. There is no risk-free level of passive smoking; even brief exposure can be harmful to your health. If possible, stay away from smokers and avoid cigarette smoke where you can

So How, Exactly, Does Extra Virgin Olive Oil Strengthen Your Body's Performance?

Extra virgin olive oil gives athletes the energy they need. In a normal adult diet, fats represent between 25% and 30% of the total energy intake. This energy intake cannot be replaced by another type of food since fatty acids are essential to maintain proper health.

That is why we must consume excellent quality fats. As you may know, if you've done a bit of prior research, we must avoid saturated fats (pastries, butter, meat, coconut, or palm oil). Instead, we should take healthier ones such as monosaturated fats like extra virgin olive oil and polyunsaturated fats (blue fish and nuts).

Whether you are training for a competition or just building your fitness and strength for wellbeing and health, your results will be influenced by the diet you eat.

The Fats In Extra Virgin Olive Oil That Contribute To A Healthy Diet

Fats are made up of fatty acids and glycerol. A fatty acid consists of a chain of carbon atoms, where each carbon atom in the chain is attached to hydrogen atoms. The number of hydrogen atoms per carbon atom determines whether the fatty acid is saturated or unsaturated and, therefore will contribute towards a healthy diet.

Saturated Fats

If a fatty acid has all the hydrogen atoms it can hold (2 per carbon atom in the chain) and all of the carbon atoms in the chain are linked by single bonds, it is described as saturated.

Saturated fats are usually solid or semi-solid at room temperature and are strongly associated with raised blood cholesterol which is why nutritionists recommend eating them as little as possible. Lard, butter, hard cheeses, whole milk, animal fats and palm and coconut oils – plus products containing them – all contain high levels of saturated fat that do not support a healthy diet.

Monounsaturated Fats Support A Healthy Diet

If a pair of carbon atoms in the fatty acid chain is linked by a double bond instead of a single bond, the fatty acid is described as monounsaturated. Fats rich in monounsaturates tend to be liquid at room temperature. Olive oil is one of the richest sources of monounsaturated fatty acids and therefore supports a healthy diet.

Monounsaturated fats—omega-6s in the case of extra virgin olive oil—are important because they help boost heart health. This is important for helping prevent health issues such as cardiovascular disease or stroke.

Polyunsaturated Fats

These contain more than one double bond and are liquid at room temperature. The main sources are vegetable oils, such as sunflower oil, corn oil, and rapeseed, but not tropical oils such as coconut, palm, and palm kernel oils.

Trans Fats

Trans fats are created when a hydrogenation process is applied to solidify oil for use in margarines or to improve a product's shelf life. This processing causes trans fats to act like saturated fats.

The following illustrates the differing fat contents of a range of products.

Fat Content Comparison

- Saturated fats
- Polyunsaturated fats
- Monounsaturated fats

Olive Oil
Sunflower Oil
Vegetable Oil
Corn Oil
Soya Bean Oil
Coconut Oil
Groundnut Oil
Margarine
Butter

What Is In 1 Tablespoon Of Extra Virgin Olive Oil?

One serving or 1 tablespoon of extra-virgin olive oil contains the following:

120 calories

10 grams of monounsaturated fat

2 grams of saturated fat

2 grams of polyunsaturated fat

1.9 milligrams of vitamin E (10 percent of Daily Value)

8.1 micrograms of vitamin K (10 percent of DV)

Not All Calories Are Created Equal

As part of maintaining a healthy diet, many people want to know how many calories are in olive oil. Research has shown that not all calories are necessarily equal.

In a famous study at Middlesex Hospital in London in the 1950s, two British researchers, Professor Alan Kekwick and Dr. Gaston L.S. Pawan, tested a series of diets on overweight patients. The patients on a high-carbohydrate diet consistently gained or sustained weight, even when given limited calories. Conversely, subjects on a high-fat diet lost considerably more weight than any of the other diets, even when provided with excess calories.

A more recent study published in The Journal of the American Medical Association also challenges the notion that a "calorie is just a calorie." Led by Cara Ebbeling, PhD, associate director, and David Ludwig, MD, director of the New Balance Foundation Obesity Prevention Center at Boston Children's Hospital, (65) the purpose of the study was to learn what kind of diet helped people maintain their new weight after successfully losing weight. The results indicated that a low-fat diet predicts weight regain, while diets featuring a moderate to the high percentage of calories from fat both increased subjects' energy expenditure and reduced the surge in their blood sugar after eating, making these diets preferable to a low-fat diet for those trying to achieve lasting weight loss.

Extra Virgin Olive Oil Nutrition

Extra virgin olive oil is nutritious. It contains modest amounts of vitamins E and K and plenty of beneficial fatty acids.

One tablespoon (13.5 grams) of olive oil contains the following:

Saturated fat:	14%
Monounsaturated fat:	73% (mostly oleic acid)
Vitamin E:	13% of the Daily Value (DV)
Vitamin K:	7% of the DV

Notably, extra virgin olive oil shines in its antioxidant content. Antioxidants are biologically active, and some of them can help fight serious diseases. The oil's main antioxidants include the anti-inflammatory oleocanthal, as well as oleuropein, a substance that protects LDL (bad) cholesterol from oxidation.

Choosing foods which are rich in healthy fats, such as Extra Virgin Olive Oil, can help improve your body's potential in many ways, including muscle recovery and increased energy levels. This is particularly good news for runners who are considering following a Mediterranean diet to improve performance. According to a recent report in Runner's World, (66) the range of foods and good fats from nuts, seeds, and extra virgin olive oil can benefit runners in several ways.

By substituting heavily processed fats in meats and refined grains with more fruit, vegetables, and fish, runners can increase their carbohydrate intake, providing the quick-burning fuel that they need.

According to Lori Russell M.S., RD, CSSD, CPT: "The boost to heart health and the cardiovascular system as a whole is the biggest benefit for athletes."

One study (67) found that following a Mediterranean Diet improved 5K running times when compared to eating a standard Western diet. The significant quantity of omega-3 fatty acids and antioxidants obtained from eating the Mediterranean way can also potentially boost endurance energy and a person's ability to stay mentally strong in performance, says Russell.

Polyphenols in Extra Virgin Olive Oil Help Muscle Recovery

The high antioxidant content in Extra Virgin Olive Oil, specifically the presence of polyphenols, can contribute to a quick recovery for athletes.

In the context of exercise performance, the primary role of polyphenols is to act as an antioxidant. Exercise causes damage to muscle cells, releasing destructive free radicals into the circulatory system. Left unchecked, these highly reactive molecules can wreak havoc on cells and various bodily processes.

Antioxidant polyphenols neutralize free radicals by converting them into more stable molecules. Therefore, if you supplement with these powerful compounds, you can reduce oxidative damage from free radicals, decreasing overall damage and promoting faster recovery.

Additionally, the Mediterranean diet can even boost the health of the families of runners, according to a 2021 study in the International Journal of Obesity. (68) Relatives of those who stuck to the diet for two years were more apt to lose weight, too.

Extra Virgin Olive Oil Protects Athletes Cardiovascular System

For an athlete, maintaining the circulatory system in good shape is a must. During an intensive sport practice, the circulatory system is put to the test. The heart rate increases and the heart pumps more blood into the aortas, which must be ready to accept the increased blood flow.

Extra virgin olive oil is one of the most important foods in a diet to prevent cardiovascular disease. The moderate intake of this oil on a day-to-day basis reduces by 30% the chance of suffering a myocardial infraction, a stroke or a cerebral infraction, and it helps to keep cholesterol at bay and avoid the formation of clots and atherosclerotic plaques.

Extra Virgin Olive Oil Helps Build Muscle

One of the polyunsaturated fats that extra virgin olive oil contains, Omega 3, is what helps to train and maintain muscles.

This is especially important for an athlete who is exposed to significant wear and tear.

Extra Virgin Olive Oil Prevents Oxidative Stress

As the intensity of the exercise increases, we consume a greater amount of oxygen but also increase our production of free radicals as a result. These radicals are responsible for fatigue but also for aging and cardiovascular diseases.

Research carried out by Jesús de la Osada, Professor of Biochemistry at the Faculty of Veterinary Medicine of the University of Zaragoza, (69) concluded that the polyphenol hydroxytyrosol, which is present in high quality extra virgin olive oil like Morocco Gold prevents oxidative stress by combating these free radicals.

The vitamin E present in best olive oil also act to counter the damaging effects that free radicals produce to our cells.

Extra Virgin Olive Oil And Sexual Wellness

As it has been with so much of traditional lore, the inherently erotic properties of olive oil lubricant were swept into the shadows by modernity and are only recently coming back to light. The ancient Egyptians, Greeks, and Romans were well-versed in the many benefits of olive oil and used it amply in sexy bedroom scenes. But as time passed, olive oil became relegated to kitchen use.

The Greeks Knew How to Live it Up

It's well known that in the ancient Greek society, all forms of physical pleasure were embraced. Rather than censoring sexual deviations, they celebrated sexuality in all its forms which can be seen in their prized art pieces.

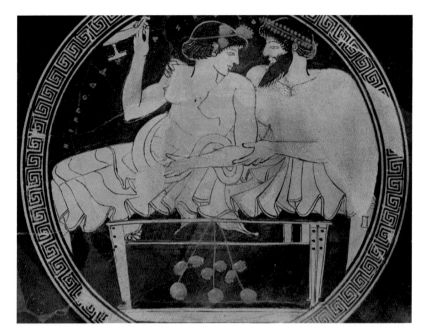

The amphorae and vases of that period depict vivid scenes of heterosexual and homosexual intercourse, group orgies, fellatio, and more. Many of them also depict other interesting details. Two amphorae can be spotted in the love making scenes, one filled with wine, the other with olive oil.

There's no question where wine fits into the scene. But the olive oil? Well, it was the choice lubricant for sexual unions.

Soak It In

Anyone who's had an essential oil massage knows how seductive olive oil can be. Rich and pungent, olive oil can be massaged deep into the pores, relaxing muscles and loosening limbs. So, when you're getting exploratory in the bedroom, you can use an all-natural olive oil lubricant. Its consistency is very close to natural lubrication, it's edible, and it makes everything glide much more sensually.

Health Boost = Sex Boost

But olive oil's role in enhancing our sex lives doesn't just begin when the lights dim. It's no secret that healthier people have healthier sexual appetites and are better equipped to appease them, too.

Olive oil lubricant enhances one's health in a plethora of ways. But there's an even more direct correlation between internal ingestion of olive oil and a fuller sex life. Olive oil boosts blood circulation throughout the body, particularly, to our elusive erogenous zones. Is it any wonder that Casanova, the most infamous lover in history, hailed from Italy, the land dripping in extra-virgin olive oil? Increased blood flow provides for more vigorous sexual experiences, and who doesn't want that?

Olive oil Lubricant: An Aid for those Advancing in Age

Olive oil plays an even more pertinent role in the bedroom as we age. Women who go through menopause often notice a painful shrinkage in vaginal areas. This can be ameliorated through internal and external olive oil massages – an exciting task to embark on either alone or with a partner.

According to sex therapist, Rita Collins, (70) "Many women think their sex lives are over after menopause, when sexual organs can morph into very unfamiliar appendages. But something as simple and pleasurable as a good olive oil massage can really put a woman back in touch with her body. I recommend women lather olive oil lubricant all over and within that region, on a regular basis, as an important step in getting back in tune with their bodies."

In a time where people will go to any extent to push the envelope and taste every form of pleasure, it's important to get back in touch with the basics. You don't need to do an illicit internet search or go to a seedy sex shop to get a case of extra virgin olive oil.

Indulge in olive oil, the aphrodisiac of the ancients, and find yourself feeling at your prime, senses open to a storehouse of physical bliss.

One For The Boys

Studies also prove that olive oil combats erectile dysfunction. The same dietary choices that lead to restricted blood flow in coronary arteries, which leads to heart attacks, and restrict blood flow to and within the penis. Research shows that those who partake in the Mediterranean diet, which includes ample amounts of olive oil, experience much less issues with erectile dysfunction.

A recent study at the University of Athens (71) showed that sticking to a Mediterranean diet with extra virgin olive oil a key constituent protects sexual performance and might be more successful long-term than Viagra.

The study involved more than 660 men with an average age of 67. They found consuming just nine tablespoons of extra virgin olive oil per week is enough to reduce the chance of impotence by 40 per cent in later life. It can also help dramatically boost testosterone levels, a key male sex hormone.

Erectile dysfunction, also known as impotence, is the inability to get and maintain an erection. But Greek researchers found a diet rich in olive oil keeps blood vessels healthy, boosting circulation to key organs.

Erectile dysfunction is a common problem which can cause problems in relationships. Impotence was reported to affect around a fifth of the study participants, significantly lower than levels in the UK among men of the same age. Around five million men in the UK alone are affected by the condition.

Causes can be psychological or physical, from stress and depression to conditions which affect blood flow, including heart disease and diabetes.

UK experts welcomed the findings. Professor Mike Wyllie, one of the scientists who developed Viagra in the 1990s, said: "The message that you can affect your sexual function by modifying lifestyle and diet is a valid one. Erectile dysfunction is usually about 80 percent a cardiovascular [heart] disease condition. Altering cardiovascular status, you get an improvement in erectile function, this study reinforces that message."

Drugs like Viagra have revolutionized the treatment, but they can have side effects - headache, back pain, and visual disturbance. And they do not work for all men and are unsuitable for men with unstable angina. They also have to be taken well in advance of sexual intercourse.

Julie Ward, Senior Cardiac Nurse at the British Heart Foundation (72) said: "It's no surprise that the Mediterranean diet which we know is beneficial to the heart and circulatory health might also benefit blood vessels elsewhere, and help men maintain healthy sexual function. Because the blood vessels in the penis are so narrow, being unable to achieve or maintain an erection can be one of the first signs of atherosclerosis the narrowing of arteries that can lead to a heart attack or stroke".

"It's crucial that any underlying medical condition, such as atherosclerosis or diabetes, is spotted early and treated to keep your heart, as well as your sex life, healthy".

This is also important for this next section!

Extra Virgin Olive Oil For Couples Trying To Conceive

Nutrition has a significant impact on fertility. To get pregnant, a couple needs a healthy egg to join to healthy sperm, which is then implanted inside the woman's uterus. Nutrition can impact the health of the egg, the health of the sperm, the production of fertility hormones which impact the timing of ovulation, the health of the uterus (and consequently the likelihood of implantation), and the growth and development of the foetus.

There are 4 key stages of support that nutrition intervention is required.

Trying To Conceive

The first stage is couples who have just started trying to conceive. The key message for these clients is the impact of nutrition on shaping their baby's future. Research suggests that pre-conception nutrition can influence genetic programming to impact a child's future weight, risk of chronic diseases, and cognitive abilities.

For example, a study by Dr Clive Petry (73) and colleagues suggests that pre-conception maternal and paternal lipid intake may impact genetic printing to influence the child's future development and metabolism. Furthermore, a Mediterranean-style diet and monounsaturated fat intake during pregnancy have been linked to decreased cardiovascular disease risk for the baby later on in life.

Dietary Conditions

Stage two is for couples with pre-existing or newly diagnosed dietary conditions, which increase the risk of infertility. Conditions include Poly Cystic Ovarian Syndrome, Endometriosis, Insulin Resistance, Inflammatory Bowel Disease, Thyroid conditions, and more. Couples with dietary conditions need to be counselled that optimal dietary management may assist in improving fertility outcomes. For example, studies suggest that endometriosis may be improved with an anti-inflammatory type of diet. Extra virgin olive oil has been found to be beneficial for immune-inflammatory diseases such as Rheumatoid Arthritis and Inflammatory Bowel Disease and may also play a protective role in endometriosis.

Current studies suggest that a Mediterranean-diet style may be beneficial for clients with Poly Cystic Ovarian Syndrome.

Assisted Reproductive Treatments

The third stage of couples requiring nutrition intervention are those undergoing Assisted Reproductive Treatments (ART). ART includes a range of procedures such as ovulation induction for women who aren't ovulating regularly and artificial insemination, where semen is transferred directly into a woman's uterus. Before moving onto In Vitro Fertilisation, solving problems utilising diet and lifestyle should be considered. For example, around 30% of fertility problems arise from male sperm health. Studies suggest that olive oil and extra virgin olive oil may help to improve semen quality and sperm functionality which may improve ART outcomes.

Secondly, optimal egg health is essential for successful ART. Inflammation in the fluid surrounding the egg impacts egg quality and decreases the chance of conception. Studies show that extra virgin olive oil helps to minimise inflammation.

Thirdly, approximately half of all embryo implantations result in a failed pregnancy. Although this can be caused by the health of the embryo, uterine receptivity is also an important factor. Women require a thick uterine lining of at least 7milimeters for implantation. Studies suggest that vitamin E supplements may help to increase the thickness of the uterine lining, although the mechanism for this remains unknown. Extra virgin olive oil is a rich dietary source of vitamin

E, and although no studies have been conducted, it is plausible that the vitamin E in extra virgin olive oil may be one of the factors contributing to its benefit in women who are trying to conceive. Furthermore, aspirin is often given to reduce inflammation. Studies show that extra virgin olive oil has significant anti-inflammatory effects.

In Vitro Fertilisation

The final stage of nutrition intervention is for couples undergoing In Vitro Fertilisation (IVF). IVF literally means 'fertilisation in a test tube'. The embryo is then transferred into the woman's uterus. Studies suggest that adherence to a Mediterranean-style diet, including the use of extra virgin olive oil may strengthen IVF outcomes. For example, a study by Dr Vujkovic (74) and colleagues found that men consuming a more Mediterranean-style diet were more likely to result in pregnancy through IVF than those consuming a less 'health conscious' dietary style which was lower in healthy oils and legumes. These results were substantiated by Dr Karayiannis (75) and colleagues, who found that a 5-point increase in the Mediterranean Diet Score resulted in a 2.7 times higher likelihood of pregnancy through IVF.

Furthermore, a diet high in olive oil and fish, and low in meat, was found to improve embryonic growth and minimise the risk of miscarriages.

Is Extra Virgin Olive Oil Safe During Pregnancy?

Before you add extra virgin olive oil to your pregnancy diet, you should know whether it is safe for you or not. Well, extra virgin olive oil is very safe for you to consume during your pregnancy and, thus, you may safely add it to your pregnancy diet. It has many benefits for pregnant woman. In fact, it is not only good for the to-be-mommy, but it also has immense benefits for the unborn baby too.

Benefits Of Extra Virgin Olive Oil for Pregnant Women

Olives are power packed with various health benefits. Apart from being rich in dietary fibre, olives are a rich source of monounsaturated fats, vitamin E, and iron. Extra virgin olive oil is very gentle on the stomach and, thus, very safe for consumption during pregnancy. Here's how it helps you and your unborn baby during pregnancy.

Vitamin E:

Olive oil may not be a high source of vitamin E. However, because of its resistance to oxidation, the quantity present offers ample benefits to a pregnant woman. Vitamin E is one of the components that help your baby to adapt better in the oxygen-filled environment soon after birth. If the mother of a premature or preterm baby consumes olive oil during the breastfeeding stage, it may help her baby to develop better.

Beneficial In Foetal Development:

If you consume olive oil during pregnancy it may greatly benefit the growth and development of your unborn baby. The substantial amounts of omega-3 fatty acids are extremely beneficial for your baby's heart. It has also been observed that consumption of olive oil during pregnancy improves brain function and development and it also improves the learning skills of your baby as he grows. Also, if a mother consumes olive oil on a regular basis during her pregnancy, it may positively impact the height and weight of her unborn baby.

Helps In Reducing Stretch Marks:

Developing stretch marks is a very common phenomenon during pregnancy, and most women may experience it. This may happen because as your baby grows, your pelvic muscles and abdomen stretch to accommodate your growing baby, which in turn may lead to stretch marks. Olive oil has been in use for a long time to overcome the problem of stretch marks during pregnancy. If you keep applying olive oil to your tummy area every day, it is possible that you may not have stretch marks during pregnancy. And even if you do develop stretch marks, they may either become light or in some cases, even disappear after regular usage. However, the only mantra that you need to follow while using olive oil for stretch marks during pregnancy is to use it on a regular basis.

Beneficial In Improving Reflexes in Babies:

It has been observed that mothers who consumed olive oil regularly during their pregnancy journey gave birth to babies who had better or improved psychomotor reflexes in comparison to women who did not consume olive oil during their pregnancy.

Helpful In Fighting Various Infections:

Pregnancy may make your immune system sluggish, and thus, may make pregnant women more susceptible to falling ill with various kinds of infections. However, including olive oil in your pregnancy diet may prove to be beneficial. This is because olive oil is a rich source of Vitamin A, which helps in building a strong immune system. This, in turn, may help in keeping various infections at bay. Also, Vitamin A is very beneficial for the eyes, and including olive oil in your pregnancy diet may not only ensure good eye-health of the would-be mother, but it may also be beneficial for fetal eye development.

It is important to remember that olive oil, like any other oil, should be consumed in moderation. You may safely consume and apply olive oil on your skin during pregnancy but refrain from going overboard with its consumption and usage. In any case, we also suggest that you get a go-ahead from your doctor before doing so, especially if you're using it for the first time. This is because every pregnancy is different, and what may be beneficial and healthy for one woman may not be for the other. Thus, your doctor may know what is best for you during your pregnancy.

In Summary

Current research suggests that extra virgin olive oil may be beneficial for fertility whether couples are trying to conceive naturally, have dietary conditions which may impact their fertility, are undergoing Assisted Reproductive Treatments or In Vitro Fertilisation.

Extra virgin olive oil is also a wonderful supplement to the diet during pregnancy.

The Effects Of A Healthy Lifestyle

Researchers from the Harvard T.H. Chan School of Public Health (76) conducted a massive study of the impact of health habits on life expectancy, using data from the well-known Nurses' Health Study (NHS) (77) and the Health Professionals Follow-up Study (HPFS) (78). This means that they had data on a huge number of people over a very long period. The NHS included over 78,000 women and followed them from 1980 to 2014. The HPFS included over 40,000 men and followed them from 1986 to 2014. This is over 120,000 participants, 34 years of data for women and 28 years of data for men.

The researchers looked at NHS and HPFS data on diet, physical activity, body weight, smoking, and alcohol consumption that had been collected from regularly administered, validated questionnaires. These five areas were chosen because prior studies have shown them to have a large impact on the risk of premature death. Here are how these healthy habits were defined and measured:

Healthy Diet

This was calculated and rated based on the reported intake of healthy foods like vegetables, fruits, nuts, whole grains, healthy fats like extra virgin olive oil and omega-3 fatty acids, and unhealthy foods like red and processed meats sugar-sweetened beverages, trans fat, and sodium.

Healthy physical activity level

This was defined as at least 30 minutes per day of moderate to vigorous activity daily.

Healthy Body Weight

Defined as a normal body mass index (BMI), which is between 18.5 and 24.9.

Smoking

There is no healthy amount of smoking. "Healthy" here meant never having smoked.

Moderate Alcohol Intake

Measured as between 5 and 15 grams per day for women and 5 to 30 grams per day for men. Generally, one drink contains about 14 grams of pure alcohol. That's 12 ounces of regular beer, 5 ounces of wine, or 1.5 ounces of distilled spirits.

Researchers also looked at data on age, ethnicity, and medication use, as well as comparison data from the National Health and Nutrition Examination Surveys and the Centres for Disease Control and Prevention's Wide-Ranging Online Data for Epidemiologic Research.

Does a healthy lifestyle make a difference?

As it turns out, healthy habits make a big difference. According to this analysis, people who met the criteria for all five habits enjoyed significantly, impressively longer lives than those who had none: 14 years for women and 12 years for men (if they had these habits at age 50). People who had none of these habits were far more likely to die prematurely from cancer or cardiovascular disease.

Study investigators also calculated life expectancy by how many of these five healthy habits people had. Just one healthy habit (and it didn't matter which one) ... *just one...* extended life expectancy by two years in men and women. Not surprisingly, the healthier habits people had, the longer their lifespan.

This is **huge.** And it confirms prior similar research — a lot of prior similar research. A 2017 study using data from the Health and Retirement Study found that people 50 and older who were normal weight, had never smoked, and drank alcohol in moderation lived on average seven years longer. A 2012 mega-analysis of 15 international studies that included over 500,000 participants found that over half of premature deaths were due to unhealthy lifestyle factors such as poor diet, inactivity, obesity, excessive alcohol intake, and smoking. And the list of supporting research goes on. (79)

CHAPTER 7.
EXTRA VIRGIN OLIVE OIL & MENTAL HEALTH

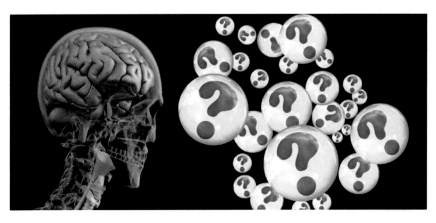

According to a study from the University of Navarra and Las Palmas de Gran Canaria (80) diet rich in extra virgin olive oil can help to protect from mental illness.

The study included 12,059 volunteers and explored the dietary determinants of stroke, coronary disease, and other disorders. The research was conducted over a period of 6 years, during which time the researchers gathered data on lifestyle factors, including diet and medical history.

The results revealed that volunteers with a high intake of trans fats had up to 48 percent increased risk of depression compared to those who did not consume those fats. In addition, the researchers also discovered that a higher intake of olive oil and polyunsaturated fats was associated with a lower risk of depression.

This is one of a wealth of studies showing how extra virgin olive oil and the Mediterranean diet are associated with lower rates of depression.

In April 2018, Dr Drew Ramsey, M.D., clinical professor of psychiatry at Columbia University (81) revealed how extra virgin olive oil impacts the brain and your overall health. Dr Ramsey listed the following key benefits of olive oil as part of a Mediterranean style diet:

Olive oil is full of healthy fats

Olive oil is rich in phytonutrients and antioxidants

Olive oil decreases the risk for depression

Olive oil decreases the risk for dementia

In 2009, Spanish researchers once again discovered that individuals who followed a Mediterranean style diet rich in olive oil, vegetables, beans, and fruit were 30 percent less likely to suffer from depression.

An Australian study named the 'SMILES' trial (82) compared participants who took part in social support groups versus those who also were counselled about healthy food choices and consumed a Mediterranean diet. After 12 weeks, nearly a third of those who also had the counselling and diet experienced remission from the depression versus only 8 percent for the support group only subjects.

According to Naturopathic Physician Vickie Modica of Seattle, Washington, "Omega-3 fatty acids, known to have an anti-inflammatory effect and thought to have a healthful impact on the nervous system, improve the symptoms of depression in multiple studies." (83).

These links between consumption of extra virgin olive oil as part of a Mediterranean diet form another layer of understanding of the proven benefits to overall cognitive function.

Extra Virgin Olive Oil Study: Aristotle University Of Thessaloniki

A new study from the Aristotle University of Thessaloniki and the Greek Association of Alzheimer's Disease and Related Disorders (84) has shown that the long-term daily consumption of extra virgin olive oil could benefit elderly people with cognitive impairments even more than previously thought.

The research, which was published in the Journal of Alzheimer's Disease, tested the effects of high-phenolic early-harvest extra virgin olive oil against moderate phenolic extra virgin olive oil and the Mediterranean diet. Until now, there is no other study that has examined in such a detailed manner the effects of extra virgin olive oil in elders with amnestic mild cognitive impairment as an effective solution.

The researchers found that high-phenolic early-harvest extra virgin olive oil served as a natural therapeutic pharmaceutical compound for older adults with amnestic mild cognitive impairment, which is considered a prodromal condition to the development of Alzheimer's disease.

Previous studies have shown the therapeutic effects of following a Mediterranean diet on improving cognitive functions while decreasing the risk of amnestic mild cognitive impairment progressing to Alzheimer's disease.

The researchers conducted a randomized prospective study to examine the high-phenolic early-harvest extra virgin olive oil and moderate phenolic extra virgin olive oil versus the Mediterranean diet in MCI. Genetic predisposition (Polymorphism in the apolipoprotein E (APOE) gene is a major genetic risk determinant of late-onset Alzheimer disease) to Alzheimer's disease was tested, and an extensive neuropsychological examination was administered at baseline and after 12 months.

Each participant was randomized and assigned one of three groups. Group 1 received the high-phenolic early-harvest extra virgin olive oil (50 mL/day); Group 2 received the moderate phenolic extra virgin olive oil (50mL/day), and 3) Group 3 received only the Mediterranean diet instructions.

The results of the study demonstrated that participants following a high-phenolic early-harvest extra virgin olive oil variation of the Mediterranean diet fared better in the 12-month follow-up performance in almost all cognitive domains of the Alzheimer's disease assessment scale-cognitive subscale, which is a scale used to understand the level of cognitive impairment caused by the disease, than adherents to the other two diets. Those patients also fared better with digit span, which focuses on the working memory activity and letter fluency.

Furthermore, adherents to the moderate phenolic extra virgin olive oil variation of the Mediterranean diet fared better on the same cognitive tests than participants in the control group, who followed a standard Mediterranean diet.

"The results of this study suggest that the long-term consumption of an extra virgin olive oil-containing diet starting at an early age provides a protective effect against Alzheimer's disease and its related disorder cerebral amyloid angiopathy," the researchers wrote.

Memory Loss & Dementia: A New Study

A new study published by The American Academy of Neurology (85), has found that adherence to the principles of The Mediterranean Diet (rich in extra virgin olive oil) may reduce your chance of developing memory loss and dementia.

Study author Tommaso Ballarini, Ph.D. explained that "Eating a diet that's high in unsaturated fats like extra virgin olive oil, fish, fruits and vegetables and low in red meat and dairy may actually protect your brain from the protein build-up that can lead to memory loss and dementia."

The study which was published in the May 2021 issue of Neurology, states that the Mediterranean diet can help prevent brain-volume shrinkage that is associated with Alzheimer's disease.

This diet traditionally consists primarily of vegetables, fruits, nuts and seeds, legumes, potatoes, whole grain foods, seafood, extra virgin olive oil, and wine in moderation.

Dietitian at Cleveland Clinic Kristin Kirkpatrick (86) told Medical News Today that this diet contributes beneficial "omega-3 fatty acids, polyphenols, specific minerals, fibre, and protein" that "may support the brain's health and protection throughout the years."

The Mediterranean Diet, Extra Virgin Olive Oil and Alzheimer's

The Study has also been well received by experts in the field of Alzheimer's Prevention. Dr Richard Isaacson, director of the Alzheimer's Prevention Clinic at Weill Cornell Medicine and New York-Presbyterian Hospital, (87) recently told CNN that "in this important study, researchers showed that it's possible to not only improve cognitive function – most specifically memory – but also reduce the risk for Alzheimer's disease pathology."

Dr Isaacson was not involved in the study but added that "for every point of higher compliance with the diet, people had one extra year less of brain aging. That is striking," CNN reported. "Most people are unaware that it's possible to take control of your brain health, yet this study shows us just that."

According to a report on the study in the National Herald, (88) The study "examined 343 people at high risk of developing Alzheimer's and compared them to 169 cognitively normal subjects," CNN reported, adding that "first, researchers tested each person's cognitive skills, including language, memory, and executive function, and used brain scans to measure brain volume. Spinal fluid from 226 participants was also tested for amyloid and tau protein biomarkers."

"Then people were asked how well they were following the Mediterranean diet," CNN reported, noting that "after adjusting for factors like age, sex and education, the study found that people who did not follow the diet closely had more signs of amyloid and tau build-up in their spinal fluid than those who did adhere to the diet."

Extra Virgin Olive Oil, The Mediterranean Diet, And Neurodegenerative Disease

According to News Medical, (89) Alzheimer's disease is the most common form of dementia in the US. It is estimated to affect approximately 5 million people in the United States alone.

The neurodegenerative disease is progressive and cannot yet be cured or reversed. Researchers from the Lewis Katz School of Medicine at Temple University (LKSOM) in Philadelphia (90), reported that extra virgin olive oil, which is the most common component in the Mediterranean Diet, boosts cognitive performance and could aid in preventing Alzheimer's. The study involved mice models that have the three components present in Alzheimer's disease, memory impairment, amyloid plaque build-up, and neurofibrillary tangles.

Beta Amyloid

Amyloid plaques are the result of the excess production and build-up of beta-amyloid, a fragment of the protein called "amyloid precursor protein." In Alzheimer's disease, these plaques build up in the spaces between neurons.

Neurofibrillary tangles are the result of twisted strands of a protein called tau. In a healthy brain, tau helps with the transportation of nutrients and other molecules that the brain cells need. In Alzheimer's disease, this protein gets tangled up inside the brain cells, which happen to be dying because essential nutrients no longer reach them.

Alzheimer's characteristics begin to develop in rodents quite early on, so in this experiment, the oil was added to the diet when the mice were 6 months old, before any symptoms could have appeared.

The mice were separated into two groups. The first were fed a regular diet, including extra virgin olive oil while the second group has no extra virgin olive oil added to their diet. The researchers evaluated the mice's cognitive abilities by administering tests for their spatial memory, working memory, and learning skills.

In terms of general appearance, no differences were noted between the two animal groups. But, when the mice were 9 months and 12 months old, the mice that had been fed the extra-virgin olive oil diet performed much better in the cognitive tests.

Lead investigator Dr. Dominica Praticò and his team also analysed the brain tissue of these mice, and the studies revealed striking differences between the appearance and functioning of the nerve cells.

Firstly, the integrity of the synapses – which are the parts of the brain cell that facilitate communication among neurons – was preserved much better in the olive oil group. Secondly, the brain tissue in the mice fed olive oil revealed a "dramatic increase" in the autophagy activation of the nerve cells. Autophagy is a process that sees nerve cells disintegrate and eliminate the toxic debris that tends to accumulate between the cells. In this experiment, the increase in autophagy led to a decrease in the amyloid plaques and tau.

Dr. Praticò says, "This is an exciting finding for us. Thanks to the autophagy activation, memory and synaptic integrity were preserved, and the pathological effects in animals otherwise destined to develop Alzheimer's disease were significantly reduced. This is a very important discovery since we suspect that a reduction in autophagy marks the beginning of Alzheimer's disease." (91)

What Is In Extra Virgin Olive Oil That Helps Protect Against Dementia?

Polyphenol Oleuropein Aglycone (OA)

Oleuropein aglycone is a glycosylated seco-iridoid, a type of bitter phenolic compound found in green olive skin, flesh, seeds, and leaves. The term oleuropein is derived from the botanical name of the olive tree, Olea Europaea. The chemical formula is: $C_{25}H_{32}O_{13}$.

Oleuropein aglycone is one of the chief polyphenols found in extra virgin olive oil. It is getting more and more global attention within the scientific and medical communities due to its biological properties including in anti-Alzheimer's disease, anti-breast cancer, anti-inflammatory, anti-hyperglycemic effect, and anti-oxidative properties.

OA is derived from the de-glycosylation of oleuropein that exists in the leaves and stones of the olive fruit during the maturation period and is obtained during the pressing of the olives.

The Effect Of Oleuropein Aglycone On Amyloidosis

Amyloidosis is the name for a group of rare but serious conditions caused by a build-up of an abnormal protein called amyloid in organs and tissues throughout the body. The build-up of amyloid protein deposits can make it difficult for the organs and tissues to work properly.

It had been reported that the aglycone form of oleuropein interferes with the build-up of a number of proteins associated with amyloidosis, particularly affecting neuro-degenerative diseases, preventing the growth of toxic oligomers (polymers with relatively few repeating units) and displaying protection against cognitive deterioration. (92)

Or in simple terms, OA provides a protective barrier between health organ cells and harmful amyloid cells.

Oleocanthal In Extra Virgin Olive Oil

The importance and uniqueness of Oleocanthal in extra virgin olive oil is that it has strong antioxidant and anti-inflammatory properties. Its anti-inflammatory action on the body is very similar to ibuprofen, one of the non-steroidal anti-inflammatory drugs most widely consumed.

Non-steroidal anti-inflammatory drugs (NSAIDS) such as aspirin, paracetamol, and ibuprofen, can be differentiated from steroids because they have far fewer secondary effects. NSAIDS have proven to have very beneficial effects in diseases that involve chronic inflammation processes, such as degenerative and neurodegenerative illnesses (Alzheimer).

Oleocanthal, one of the key polyphenols in high quality extra virgin olive oils, could help to prevent and treat Alzheimer's Disease, according to new research. Researchers at the University of Louisiana-Monroe (93) have identified the potential benefits of an oral supplement containing Oleocanthal.

The latest research, published in Nutrients, investigated the interaction between oleocanthal and the complementary peptide C3a receptor 1 (c3AR1), which is also involved in other types of neurogenerative diseases.

Khalid El Sayed, a pharmaceutical and toxicological sciences professor at the University of Louisiana- Monroe, and co-author of the study said:

"The complement system is an important element of the innate immune system, which enhances the antibodies and phagocytic cells to clear damaged cells and pathogenic microbes. The oleocanthal modulation [regulation] of C3AR1 is a very important finding that will direct future studies of oleocanthal as a plausible nutraceutical for prevention and modulation of pre-Alzheimer's disease neurodegenerative conditions."

El Sayed goes on to say that consumption of extra virgin olive oil is understood to have a contribute to reduced risk of cognitive diseases among Mediterranean nations, compared to other European and American populations.

"Oleocanthal has been reported to show promising activities against the markers of neurodegenerative insults that lead to cognitive diseases *in vitro* and in animal models."

Simple Diet Tweaks That Could Cut Your Alzheimer's Risk

Dubbed the "MIND" diet, short for Mediterranean-DASH (Dietary Approaches to Stop Hypertension) Intervention for Neurodegenerative Delay, this eating pattern recommends natural plant-based foods while limiting red meat, saturated fat, and sweets. Observational studies suggest the diet can reduce the risk of developing Alzheimer's disease by up to 53 percent as well as slow cognitive decline and improve verbal memory.

Researchers developed the diet by looking at the Mediterranean and DASH diets, then focusing on the foods with the most compelling findings in dementia prevention. Vegetables, especially leafy greens, rose to the top and, of course, the cornerstone of the Mediterranean diet, extra virgin olive oil.

Researchers then tracked detailed eating logs in an older adult population for an average of 4.5 years to uncover trends among the diets of those who developed dementia versus those who didn't. Their discovery: Older adults whose diets most closely resembled the pattern laid out in the MIND diet had brains as sharp as people 7.5 years younger. That's a substantial difference, since delaying dementia by just five years has been suggested to cut the cost and prevalence of the disease in half.

Extra Virgin Olive Oil Can Delay The Onset Of Parkinson's Disease.

New research has linked adherence to a Mediterranean and MIND Diet (94) to later onset of Parkinson's Disease, according to the International Parkinson and Movement Disorder Society.

The research was conducted by the University of British Columbia (UBC) and compared two diets: the Mediterranean and Mediterranean-DASH Intervention for Neurodegenerative Delay (MIND) diets. The UBC study included 225 participants with Parkinson's disease and 156 control participants. The Mediterranean diet had a more positive correlation with men and the MIND diet with women in the group.

The study concluded that a strong correlation was found between the age of onset of Parkinson's Disease and dietary habits, suggesting that nutritional strategies, including high quality extra virgin olive oil, may be an effective tool to delay PD onset by up to 17.4 years for women and 8.4 years for men.

Dr. Silke Appel-Cresswell, neurologist, UBC Faculty of Medicine said: "The study shows individuals with Parkinson's disease have a significantly later age of onset if their eating pattern closely aligns with the Mediterranean-type diet." (95)

Both diets include extra virgin olive oil, vegetables, seafood, peas, beans, lentils, and wine in moderation. A major factor identified in helping to combat the disease is the presence of antioxidant polyphenols. Researchers also cited Oleuropein found in extra virgin olive oil as having cytoprotective properties for brain cells, which prevents compounds associated with Parkinson's disease from damaging them.

Parkinson's disease is known to affect around 1 million people in the USA, with around 60,000 diagnosed with the disease every year.

Silke Appel-Cresswell continued: "There is a lack of medications to prevent or delay Parkinson's disease, yet we are optimistic that this new evidence suggests nutrition could potentially delay the onset of the disease,"

Plant-Based Diet Has 'Significant Impact On The Risk Of Stroke'

A new study has revealed links between a 'healthy' plant-based diet, including foods containing polyphenols, flavonoids, and dietary fibre, and a lowered risk of stroke. The findings in the research, published online in Neurology, indicated that plant-based foods are rich in nutrients, such as polyphenols, that may reduce the risk for cardiovascular disease. Scientists have indicated that ingestion of these health-giving nutrients could be the mechanism through which a plant-based diet reduces the risk for stroke.

However, this most recent study (looking at data from over 200,000 men and women), found that maintaining a healthy plant-based diet is associated with a lower risk for both total stroke and ischemic stroke. According to study co-author Megu Baden, PhD, in the Department of Nutrition at the Harvard T.H. Chan School of Public Health:

"We found that those following this [plant-based] diet had 10% lower stroke risk. This was especially true when we take the quality of food into consideration." (96)

As explained in Medscape by Erica Camargo Faye, MD, PhD, a stroke neurologist at the Massachusetts General Hospital and an instructor in neurology at Harvard Medical School, Boston, Massachusetts:

"There is a large body of literature supporting the concept that the Mediterranean diet, DASH diet, and diets rich in fruits and vegetables reduce the risk of stroke," said Faye. "This study adds to these findings, demonstrating that the quality of plant-based diets also has a significant impact on the risk of stroke." (97)

Further Evidence That Extra Virgin Olive Oil Reduces Risk Of Stroke

A previous study carried out in France suggests that consuming olive oil may help prevent a stroke in older people. The research was published in the online issue of Neurology, the medical journal of the American Academy of Neurology. (98)

"Our research suggests that a new set of dietary recommendations should be issued to prevent stroke in people 65 and older," said study author Cécilia Samieri, PhD, with the University of Bordeaux and the National Institute of Health and Medical Research (INSERM) in Bordeaux, France. "Stroke is so common in older people, and olive oil would be an inexpensive and easy way to help prevent it."

For the study, researchers looked at the medical records of 7,625 people ages 65 and older from three cities in France: Bordeaux, Dijon, and Montpellier. Participants had no history of stroke. Olive oil consumption was categorized as "no use," "moderate use" such as using olive oil in cooking or as dressing or with bread, and "intensive use," which included using olive oil for both cooking and as dressing or with bread. Samieri said the study participants mainly used extra virgin olive oil, as that is 98 percent of what is available in France.

After a little over five years, there were 148 strokes.

After considering diet, physical activity, body mass index, and other risk factors for stroke, the study found that those who regularly used olive oil for both cooking and as dressing had a 41 percent lower risk of stroke compared to those who never used olive oil in their diet (1.5 percent in six years compared to 2.6 percent).

CHAPTER 8.
EXTRA VIRGIN OLIVE OIL & COVID

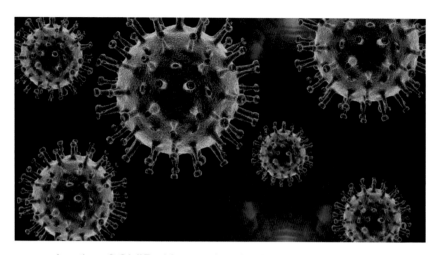

As the COVID-19 pandemic lingers, researchers have found associations between certain lifestyle factors and a person's risk of getting infected. While it has already been established that those with Type II diabetes and a high body mass index (BMI) are at greater risk of experiencing hospitalizations and other severe complications related to COVID-19, they are also at greater risk of getting a symptomatic infection in the first place. That is the finding of a recent study conducted by roocarchers at the University of Maryland School of Medicine that was recently published in the journal PLoS ONE. (99)

Using data from the UK Biobank of 500,000 British volunteers over age 40, the researchers examined health factors in those who tested positive for COVID-19 and compared them to those who tested negative. They found that those who had positive COVID-19 test results were more likely to be obese or have Type II diabetes. Those who tested negative were more likely to have high levels of "good" HDL cholesterol and be at a healthy weight with a normal body mass index (BMI).

"Certain baseline cardiometabolic factors appear to either protect a person from COVID-19 infection while others make a person more vulnerable to infection," said study author Charles Hong, MD, PhD, professor of medicine and director of cardiology research at the University of Maryland School of Medicine. "But this study wasn't designed to determine what factors actually cause COVID-19 infections. These are statistical associations that point to the importance of a healthy functioning immune system for protecting against COVID-19 infection."

He and his colleagues controlled for potential confounding factors like socioeconomic status, age, gender, and ethnicity.

"Our findings point to some healthy measures people can take to help potentially lower their risk of COVID-19 infection," Dr. Hong said. "Controlling body weight is very important during this time, and measures to increase HDL levels like regular exercise and a diet rich in monounsaturated fats like extra virgin olive oil and avocados might be helpful too." (100)

Why The Best Extra Virgin Olive Oil May Help Protect Against Covid

A common feature for many patients that get severe COVID is serious lung damage caused by an overly vigorous immune response. This is characterised by the creation of lots of inflammatory products called cytokines.

Extra virgin olive oil has been shown to reduce levels of cytokine in the body, which in turn can reduce both the symptoms associated with COVID-19 and their severity. Cytokines are small proteins that are crucial in controlling the growth and activity of other immune system cells and blood cells. When released, they signal the immune system to do its job. Cytokines affect the growth of all blood cells and other cells that help the body's immune and inflammation responses.

Although cytokines are an important component of our immune system, too many of these can lead to what is known as a 'cytokine storm'. As reported in The Lancet, this is essentially an overreaction of our immune system, which can have a seriously detrimental impact on COVID-19 sufferers (101) and, in some cases, lead to fatality. This is because cytokine storms reduce the amount of oxygen circulating in our blood, causing fluid build-up in the lungs and lead to life-threatening breathing difficulties.

Inflammation Can Go Too Far

Many white blood cells create cytokines, but specialised cells called monocytes and macrophages seem to be some of the biggest culprits in generating cytokine storms. When properly controlled, these cells are a force for good that can detect and destroy threats, clear and repair damaged tissue, and bring in other immune cells to help.

However, in severe COVID the way monocytes and macrophages work misfires. And this is particularly true in patients with diabetes and obesity.

Glucose Fuels Damage

Diabetes, if not controlled well, can result in high levels of glucose in the body. A recent study (102) showed that, in COVID, macrophages and monocytes respond to high levels of glucose with worrying consequences.

The virus that causes COVID, SARS-CoV-2, needs a target to latch onto to invade our cells. Its choice is a protein on the cell surface called ACE2. Glucose increases the levels of ACE2 present on macrophages and monocytes, helping the virus infect the very cells that should be helping to kill it.

Cytokines, small proteins released by several immune cells, play a key role in directing the immune response. (103)

Once the virus is safely inside these cells, it causes them to start making lots of inflammatory cytokines – effectively kick-starting the cytokine storm. And the higher the levels of glucose, the more successful the virus is at replicating inside the cells – essentially, the glucose fuels the virus.

But the virus isn't done yet. It also causes the virally infected immune cells to make products that are very damaging to the lung, such as reactive oxygen species. And on top of this, the virus reduces the ability of other immune cells – lymphocytes – to kill it.

Obesity also causes high levels of glucose in the body and, like diabetes, affects macrophage and monocyte activation. (104) Research has shown that macrophages from obese individuals are an ideal place for SARS-CoV-2 to thrive.

Inflammation: A Key Factor That Explains Vulnerability To Severe COVID

The severity of COVID-19 can vary hugely. In some, it causes no symptoms at all, and in others it's life-threatening, with some people particularly vulnerable to its very severe impacts.

The virus disproportionately affects men and people who are older and who have conditions such as diabetes and obesity. In the UK and other western countries, ethnic minorities have also been disproportionately affected.

While many factors contribute to how severely people are affected, including access to healthcare, occupational exposure, and environmental risks such as pollution, it is becoming clear that for some of these at-risk groups, it's the response of their immune system – inflammation – that explains why they get so sick.

Specifically, we're seeing that the risks associated with diabetes, obesity, age, and sex are all related to the immune system functioning irregularly when confronted by the virus.

Other Risks Tied To Inflammation

The same sort of inflammatory profile that diabetes and obesity cause is also seen in some older people (those over 60 years). This is due to a phenomenon known as inflammageing.

Inflammageing is characterised by having high levels of pro-inflammatory cytokines. It's influenced by several factors, including genetics, the microbiome (the bacteria, viruses, and other microbes that live inside and on you), and obesity.

Many older people also have fewer lymphocytes – the very cells that can specifically target and destroy viruses.

This all means that for some older people, their immune system is not only poorly equipped to fight off an infection, but it is also more likely to lead to a damaging immune response. Having fewer lymphocytes also means vaccines may not work as well, which is crucial to consider when planning a future COVID vaccine campaign.

Another puzzle that has been worrying researchers is why men seem so much more vulnerable to COVID. One reason is that cells in men seem to be more readily infected by SARS-CoV-2 than women. The ACE2 receptor that the virus uses to latch onto and infect cells is expressed much more highly in men than women. Men also have higher levels of an enzyme called TMPRSS2 that promotes the ability of the virus to enter the cells.

Immunology is also offering some clues on the sex difference. It's long been known that men and women differ in their immune responses, and this is true in COVID.

A recent pre-print (research that has not yet been reviewed) has tracked and compared the immune response to

SARS-CoV-2 in men and women over time. It found that men were more likely to develop atypical monocytes that were profoundly pro-inflammatory and capable of making cytokines typical of a cytokine storm. Women also tended to have a more robust T cell response, which is needed for effective virus killing. However, increased age and having a higher body mass index reversed the protective immune effect in women.

Studies like these highlight how different people are. The more we understand these differences and vulnerabilities, the more we can consider how best to treat each patient. Data like these also highlight the need to consider variation in immune function and include people of varied demographics in drug and vaccine trials. (105)

Extra Virgin Olive Oil To Fight Inflammation

Polyphenol rich olive oil fights inflammation in the body and can regulate muscle damage or chemicals that cause inflammation. As inflammation is related to various other diseases, polyphenols in extra virgin olive oil help to fight these diseases including cardiovascular problems.

Inflammation is a natural response to potential dangers and damage to organs in our body, however it can become self-perpetuating leading to long-term problems. There are 2 types of inflammatory diseases, acute and chronic.

Poor diet can contribute to long-term chronic inflammatory diseases. A healthy diet, like the Mediterranean diet, including extra virgin olive oil like Morocco Gold, can help combat inflammatory diseases.

Inflammation is a critical response to potential danger signals and damage in organs in our body. In diseases such as rheumatoid arthritis, lupus, ulcerative colitis, Crohn's disease, and others, the immune system turns against the bodies' organs. These painful and, in some cases, progressively debilitating conditions can take a toll on people's quality of life and create both societal and economic burdens.

The inflammatory process in the body serves an important function in the control and repair of injury. Commonly referred to as the inflammatory cascade, or simply inflammation, it can take two basic forms, acute and chronic. Acute inflammation, part of the immune response, is the body's immediate response to injury or assault due to physical trauma, infection, stress, or a combination of all three. Acute inflammation helps to prevent further injury and facilitates the healing and recovery process.

When inflammation becomes self-perpetuating, however, it can result in chronic or long-term inflammation. This is known as chronic inflammation, and lasts beyond the actual injury, sometimes for months or even years. It can become a problem itself and require medical intervention to control or stop further inflammation-mediated damage.

Chronic inflammation can affect all parts of the body. Inflammation can also be a secondary component of many diseases. For example, in atherosclerosis, or hardening of the arteries where, chronic inflammation of blood vessel walls can result in plaque build-up in the arteries, arterial or vascular blockages, and heart disease. Chronic inflammation also plays a significant role in other diseases and conditions, including chronic pain, poor sleep quality, obesity, physical impairment, and overall decreased quality of life.

The polyphenols Oleuropein Aglycone and Oleocanthal within extra virgin olive oil can help combat inflammatory diseases.

Extra Virgin Olive Oil Can Contribute To Reduced Levels of Anxiety

New research linking weight gain during lockdown with increased levels of anxiety may lead to greater dietary interventions in any future pandemics.

According to a new study published in the European Journal Of Clinical Nutrition (106), proven associations between diet quality and anxiety may result in a preventative dietary policy, particularly relevant given the increased risk of adverse COVID-19 outcomes associated with obesity.

The study concluded: "These findings suggest the need for routine and continuous surveillance of the nutritional and psychological consequences of outbreaks as part of healthcare preparedness efforts. Primary care physicians should refer people with high anxiety or substantial weight gain during the pandemic to appropriate mental health and dietetic treatment, as needed."

Mediterranean Diets, consisting of fruit, vegetables, fish, and extra virgin olive oil, has long been associated with boosting mental health. The well-documented 2017 SMILES trial (107) showed that following a modified Mediterranean diet for three months had reduced their depressive symptoms.

"It was the first clinical trial to say: 'If we take people who have moderate to severe clinical depression and we help them to improve their diet, will that improve their depression?' And we found that it did,", explained Professor Felice Jacka, director of the Food and Mood Centre at Deakin University and author of the study.

A further study from PREDIMED (108) which listed extra virgin olive oil in the title, showed that eating a Mediterranean Diet both protected the heart health of its participants but also reduced the incidence of depressive symptoms.

Research from this study also highlighted secondary benefits to sleep quality of those who followed the Mediterranean Diet – which is also known to be a great mood booster.

What Is The Link Between Extra Virgin Olive Oil And Mental Health?

The answer to this question lies within the trillions of live bacteria that live in our digestive system. When out of balance, these microbes inside our gut have been linked to obesity, autoimmune disorders, asthma, allergies, and diabetes. It's quite a list, isn't it?!

In addition, links have been found between depression, anxiety, and mood disorders, and imbalanced gut microbiota. So, looking after our gut health maybe even more important than we previously thought.

There is also a well-known link between our digestive system and our central nervous system, commonly referred to as the "gut-brain axis". Ever experienced a feeling of butterflies in your stomach when anxiety levels are raised? Well, that could very well be your "gut-brain axis" in action!

Extra virgin olive oil is packed full of anti-inflammatory compounds, which, according to Naturopathic Physician Vickie Modica of Seattle, Washington, can "have a healthful impact on the nervous system, improve the symptoms of depression in multiple studies."

Long Covid and Extra Virgin Olive Oil

Patients suffering from the symptoms of Long Covid are involved in a new trial of a supplement made from polyphenols from olives and flavonoids from oranges.

The clinical trial, which is being conducted by the Regional University of Malaga, (109) will explore how polyphenols present in extra virgin olive oil could alleviate the symptoms of Long Covid due to their antioxidant and anti-inflammatory properties.

The Endothelyx 45 supplement will be given to patients who have passed the acute phase of the disease but continue to struggle with symptoms such as chronic fatigue, joint pain, and memory loss. The research aims to study the effects of the supplement on endothelial cells, which are found in the inner lining of the arteries and play a key role in cardiovascular health.

Emerging scientific knowledge research suggests that Covid-19 attacks the body by causing inflammation and oxidative stress in the endothelial cells. Polyphenols act as an antioxidant, minimizing free radicals in the body. Antioxidants affect human health in various ways, from improving body functions and digestion to skincare. Antioxidants can also fight off cell damage in the body, enhancing the body's capability to fight off any diseases.

A separate trial is being carried out by the University Hospital of Jaén, (110) in which another food supplement containing polyphenols from olives is being administered to patients with mild or moderate Covid-19 symptoms to study its efficacy in preventing the illness from progressing to the acute stages.

Why Extra Virgin Olive Oil Benefits Your Immune System

Regular consumption of extra virgin olive oil as part of a balanced Mediterranean Diet is one of eight recommended steps to help support a healthy immune system. But why, exactly, does the best quality extra virgin olive oil have such a powerful effect on our immune system?

According to Ahmad Alkhatib, a researcher at Teesside University Center for Public Health: "Olive oil, especially extra virgin olive oil, contains monounsaturated fatty acids and several polyphenols including oleuropein and hydroxytyrosol.

These have several antioxidative and anti-inflammatory properties, which can be linked with significant antiviral and antibacterial potential." (111)

"Oleuropein has shown potential antiviral activity against the respiratory syncytial virus, a common upper respiratory infection virus. This effect has been attributed to the antioxidative property of elenolic acid, the main fragment in oleuropein."

Extra virgin olive oil is identified as one of the key foods in the Mediterranean diet with excellent antiviral superpowers. Vegetables, fish, nuts, herbs and seeds are all known to produce similar effects. This is due to the presence of polyphenols, flavonoids, sterols and unsaturated fatty acids all of which contribute to these powerful properties.

CHAPTER 9.
OLIVE OIL BEAUTY & WELLBEING

One of the favourite natural beauty products of the beauty queen Cleopatra was extra virgin olive oil. Over the last decade, many beauticians are advocating the use of olive oil due to its many beauty benefits, but the fact is that this natural ingredient has been used on the body for centuries. It was commonly used in Egypt as a cosmetic, and it is still being used in the cosmetic industry today.

Olive oil is packed with vitamins, minerals, and natural fatty acids. It can even be used on sensitive skin. Olive oil is a potent natural ingredient in anti-aging skincare beauty products. Due to its high-level antioxidant contents, it prevents skin aging and the occurrence of wrinkles and fine lines on the skin. In a nutshell, it can guard, nourish, and rejuvenate skin.

Olive oil contains vitamins E and A that helps in elongating your youth, hydrating skin, and sustaining skin's elasticity and softness. Moreover, it helps to regenerate skin cells. The list of beauty benefits of olive oil on skin, hair, face, nails, and body is very long and makes it a superb natural beauty product.

Using Extra Virgin Olive Oil For Skin

The secret of extra virgin olive oil as a natural, effective moisturizer was known by the ancient Greeks and Romans. They knew that this natural oil, all by itself, was all they needed to use to keep their skin looking young. What they will not have known is that the chemical composition of extra virgin olive oil is very close to that of human skin. Because of this similarity, your skin may absorb olive oil more easily than it would a commercial moisturizer. It also helps lock in moisture in the skin. Simply put some in your hands and start rubbing it over your entire body and face.

Extra virgin olive oil is considered a tonic for the skin. The antioxidants Vitamin E and monounsaturated fatty acids in extra virgin olive oil are very beneficial for the skin.

We have all suffered in some way due to the Covid pandemic, and many have reported accelerated signs of physical or mental aging as a result.

But did you know that some simple steps, including the adoption of a Mediterranean diet rich in unsaturated fats such as extra virgin olive oil, can help your body combat ill health and stress?

Last year, research from the University of Navarra in Pamplona, Spain (112) studied the effect of diet on telomeres or segments of DNA at the ends of each chromosome that become shorter every time a cell divides. If they get too short to do their job, the cells will cease working properly, and, in turn, we will age more quickly. *

The research reported that from the 900 people aged over 57 studied- those who ate the most ultra-processed foods had twice the incidence of short telomeres than others, and therefore an increased rate of aging.

In contrast, research last year in the journal Advances in Nutrition (113) reported that the more people adhere to a Mediterranean diet, the longer is their telomeres.

It comes as no surprise that we have turned in abundance to a greater reliance on processed junk food during lockdown, which, according to the research stated above, can cause body-wide inflammation that damages telomeres and DNA.

The advice from the combined findings of this research therefore suggests that incorporating more vegetables, fruit, nuts, beans, cereals, grains, fish, and unsaturated fats in your diet as well as reducing your intake of meat and dairy can help protect the role of these vital telomeres.

The high percentage of unsaturated fat and vitamins A and E are helpful in preventing sun damage also work on the outside to soothe and replenish, particularly sensitive skin. It is also pure and unmixed with anything but water, unlike other oils.

There is only one ingredient in extra virgin olive oil...olive oil. If you go into your bathroom and check out the ingredient list on your moisturizer, you will see a range of chemical additives. Why use something with that many ingredients when you can just use a naturally occurring extra virgin olive oil? From your head to your toes, extra virgin olive oil can be used in a variety of skincare routines that provide an all-natural alternative to soaps and creams that contain harsh chemicals.

What Makes Extra Virgin Olive Oil So Good For The Skin? Polyphenols

Polyphenols are a key component in extra virgin olive oil and are one of the best health-enhancing benefits of the oil. Many of the fruits and vegetables we consume contain many compounds critical for life. One such type of compound is known as antioxidants. Polyphenols are powerful antioxidants.

Why are antioxidants so important for our health? Oxidation is a natural process our cells use to create energy from the oxygen we inhale. As energy is being produced in our cells, some oxygen molecules (known as oxygen free radicals or reactive oxygen species) are produced as a by-product of these processes. These oxygen free radicals can damage your cells and DNA when in high concentration. Continuous damage by oxygen free radicals most often termed oxidative stress, can lead to various conditions, including wrinkling associated with age.

Extra Virgin Olive Oil Prevents Signs of Aging

One of the top health benefits of extra virgin olive oil is its antioxidants that can improve your health inside and out. The antioxidant hydroxytyrosol helps to improve your skin, including preventing aging, according to olive oil expert Paul Vossen. With its Vitamin E properties, extra virgin olive oil protects the skin from harmful damage and can help prevent wrinkles and fine lines.

Here are some other ways that you can use extra virgin olive oil as part of your beauty and wellness routine.

Olive Oil Bath

In 2006 Sophia Loren, at the age of 72 was voted World's Most Naturally Beautiful Woman. In an interview, she was asked what her secret is, and she said the "Love of Life" and "Olive Oil." Loren takes olive oil baths and uses them as a moisturizer. This would make sense that she was driven to do this because her ancient Roman ancestors did as well. Bathing in olive oil was a sign of power and wealth.

Because the oil's fat composition is very similar to that of human skin, it rarely causes allergic reactions. In addition, it's absorbed quickly and helps lock in moisture in the skin. The high percentage of unsaturated fat and vitamins A and E, helpful in preventing sun damage, also work on the outside to soothe and replenish particularly sensitive skin. It is also pure and unmixed with anything but water, unlike other oils.

To prepare the olive oil bath, just add 5 tablespoons of extra virgin olive oil into your bathtub, and you are done! (you can add more if you like). This simple yet amazing beauty secret can make your skin soft and very smooth.

Extra Virgin Olive Oil Soften Cuticles

Protect your nail cuticles from drying and ripping in the cold winter months and soften them up with some extra virgin olive oil. By caring for your cuticles, you can also strengthen your nails and improve the softness of your hands, all at the same time with one natural ingredient.

Preventing Sunburn

We love the sun, but sometimes, our skin doesn't. If you've spent a little too much time in the sun and have a resulting painful sunburn, the antioxidant properties in extra virgin olive oil can help alleviate that painful sting. These antioxidant properties also could reduce potential UVB-ray skin tumours. Just be sure to put your extra virgin olive oil on after your time in the sun, not before. With the protection from free radicals, extra virgin olive oil provides a great after-sun care routine.

Olive Oil As A Moisturizer

Extra virgin olive oil's soothing properties make it a great option for an all-natural moisturizer. For especially dry skin, you can massage some oil on your slightly damp skin. Doing so not only adds much-needed smoothness to your hands it also protects your skin from further damage. Be sure not to use too much oil on your face, which may lead to clogged pores. For a great hand scrub, mix sugar and oil together to make a natural exfoliant that keeps your hands super smooth.

For itchy, dry skin, the compound found in extra virgin olive oil called oleocanthal calms and soothes irritated skin. When regular body lotion isn't enough, slathering on some extra virgin olive oil can be a great way to get back that silky smooth skin. You need not depend on expensive body lotion to make your skin look beautiful. Immediately after you have the shower, apply and light layer of extra virgin olive oil on your skin.

Extra virgin olive oil penetrates deeply to regenerate cells and soften the tissue. This helps to retain the moisture and make this skin smooth and soft. Use the oil lavishly on elbows, knees, and feet as these areas are drier than the rest of the skin.

Body Scrub

You can use olive oil on the skin for a body scrub. Apply the extra virgin olive oil on all over your skin and then scrub the skin with sugar or coarse salt. You will find several body scrubs with olive oil

Facial Cleansing

Olive oil is great for cleansing the face and skin. The excess skin oil (sebum) and dirt that clogs the skin pores will get dissolved in the olive oil that you will apply to your face. Apply the olive oil on facial skin and massage the face with your fingers in a circular motion for 5 minutes. Then you can then wash off the oil from the face using warm water. This treatment may be good if you have oily skin.

A Natural Makeup Remover

It serves a dual purpose. While gently removing makeup nourishes your skin as well. Just put a dab of olive oil on a cotton ball or pad and gently wipe out all the makeup from your face. If you want to remove heavy makeup, first massage olive oil gently all over your face, and then wipe away all the makeup with a soft washcloth soaked with warm water. If needed, repeat it a couple of times and make sure to do it gently – never rub your skin harshly. Rinse your face with warm water followed by a splash with cold water. Cold water will not only close your skin pores but stimulate blood circulation as well.

Exfoliation

You can make an exfoliating facial scrub using a mixture of 1 tablespoon olive oil and ½ teaspoon sea salt/sugar; apply the mixture on the face and rinse the face with warm water after 10 minutes.

Treating Acne

Olive oil contains natural antibacterial properties that can effectively reduce the flare-ups on the skin caused by acne. The anti-inflammatory elements in olive oil reduce swelling and pain that occur with the outburst of pimples.

Shaving Lubricant

Using olive oil is an excellent lubricant for shaving both body and facial hair. Of course, it may create little stickiness and less glide, but the clean-up is perfect, and olive oil also makes your skin smooth after the share. Olive oil is also a good substitute for after-shave lotion.

Strengthen Nails With Olive Oil

A warm olive oil bath for nails is an excellent way to strengthen them. It takes only 5 or 10 minutes. Just soak your nails in slightly warmed-up olive oil (not too hot, just room temperature). Do this treatment once or twice a week and enjoy strong, shiny, and healthy nails!

Olive Oil Eye Cream

Yes, you can use olive oil as an eye cream. It will nourish the tender skin around your eyes and soften fine lines. Gently dab some olive oil under your eyes before bedtime or in the morning. Keep your olive oil eye cream in the fridge and enjoy refreshing, vitamin-filled beauty treatment.

Olive Oil Homemade Face Masks

Mix one egg yolk with a tablespoon of olive oil (you can also add a teaspoon of lemon juice if you want to whiten and brighten your skin, as lemon juice is rich in antioxidants and especially vitamin C). Apply this mixture to your clean face for 5 -10 minutes; rinse with warm, then cold water (cold water will help to close pores). This olive oil homemade face mask can be used for normal or dry skin types, it will nourish and soften your skin, adding a wonderful glow.

You Are What You Eat

There is evidence to suggest that some foods containing saturated fats can lead to inflammation and, in turn, several skin conditions, including acne, eczema, and rosacea. In addition, studies have shown that refined carbohydrates, including bread, pasta, and sugary treats, have been linked to acne.

Fibre is essential for keeping your bowel movements regular, lowering bad cholesterol, and feeling full for longer. On top of that, maintaining a healthy gut is a shortcut to healthy skin. Poor gut health has been linked to increased inflammation, which in turn can exacerbate skin conditions like acne and dryness.

What's more, fibre helps your digestive system better absorb nutrients and antioxidants that may help your skin and overall health. If you've been loading up on nutrients like vitamin C and collagen while skimping on fibre, your skin might not be getting the full benefits. Prebiotic fibre which can be found in foods like bananas, artichokes, onions, garlic, and whole grains is best for supporting a healthy microbiome and positively impacting skin.

Although some oily foods may mess with your skin, it's important to incorporate some healthy fats and oils into your diet. And, The Mediterranean diet provides a great guide to influence your choices of healthy fats and oils, especially quality polyphenol-rich extra virgin olive oils which can help to keep your skin healthy and glowing.

Extra Virgin Olive Oil For Hair

According to guidance in Healthline (114), using olive oil for hair care routines can add softness and strength by penetrating the hair shaft and preserving moisture. By smoothing the outer cuticle of the hair, olive oil can add shine to the appearance of the hair.

But how does it compare with coconut oil? According to a report by idiva.com (115) coconut oil has a rich, thick texture and is super-absorbent, but this can have its disadvantages when it comes to hair. For those of us with frizzy, damaged, or particularly thick hair, olive oil can be a great option for pre-shampoo massage oil. It can soften the texture of the hair and make it a lot silkier than coconut oil does, as well as be more moisturizing.

According to Idiva, the ideal approach could be a little bit of both. So, if you have a special occasion coming up and a little bit of extra time to prepare, a combination of coconut oil and olive oil for your hair and skin could be a winning option.

Cipriana Quann And TK Wonder Use Extra Virgin Olive Oil For Haircare Overnight

Meet identical twins Cipriana Quann and TK Wonder, the girls that make heads turn when they walk the streets. A while ago, the now fashion models hated their luscious hair: "I was beginning to actually hate my hair and seeing it as a huge obstacle," Cipriana said. But as time passed, they decided to stop straightening it, and start embracing it. Which eventually led the photo models to be recognized as the queens of natural hair, bringing Instagram envy all around the world.

But the sisters aren't just pretty faces. Along with their friend Nikisha Brunson, they are also the girls behind the natural hair blog "Urban Bush Babes." "I think it came to a point where it was derogatory toward people who wore their natural hairstyles, and there was a certain stigma around people who wore their hair natural or in an Afro," TK Wonder said. "It was about breaking down stereotypes and derogatory perceptions that people had about natural hair." Now, whatever the twins do, they do it with ambition, confidence, passion, and, of course, great hair.

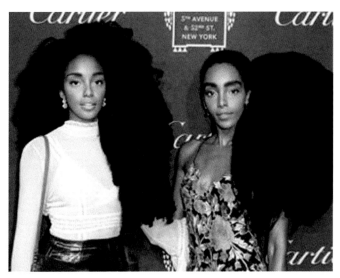

Cipriana said, "I have been natural for almost eight years now. The journey was a long one, but to keep it short, I just became more comfortable in my natural identity. After years and years of modelling and struggling with my physical image regarding my hair of trying to mould it into someone else's idea of their "ideal beauty," I'd just had enough! I wanted to represent tho kind of heauty I felt most comfortable with and idolized when I was younger, which was my mother's Image.

I was done with masking my identity to represent a false beauty to please the standards of others. Beauty is in the eye of the beholder, and at the end of the day, I realized the most important beholder was me".

Cipriana says, "My hair continually stays in loose twists no matter what the style, so I will take down my loose twists at night from whatever style I am wearing now and braid it into six or seven large braids or Bantu knots, placing a little extra virgin olive oil on the strands as I braid. Then I wrap it with a silk scarf.

In the morning, it just consists of undoing my night-time routine and placing back into my updo style.

Miranda Kerr Uses Olive Oil For Hair Mask

Continuing down the haircare path, Miranda Kerr revealed to Elle (116) that she uses olive oil as a DIY hair mask. I sleep with olive oil in my hair once a week as a treatment, it nourishes the scalp and leaves my hair super shiny," Kerr said.

Celebrity Hair Stylist Recommends Hot Olive Oil Hair Treatment

Speaking to Good Housekeeping, (118) celebrity hairstylist Gabrielle Corney recommended using a hot olive oil treatment.

"You can also add olive oil to a deep conditioner to really soften the hair. Or apply a small amount of it to the hair and scalp as a daily styling shot of moisture as well as for adding some lustre and shine. Used alongside a healthy hair care regime, olive oil for hair brings plenty of good to the table. But remember, a little goes a long way. Too much of it can weigh the hair down!"

Olive Oil And Hair Growth

Olive oil in hair does encourage hair growth: it reduces hair loss by preventing the hormone dihydrotestosterone, or DHT, from binding to the scalp, and olive oil contains antifungal properties and moisturizers that stimulate hair production, too. Olive oil helps make hair roots stronger and contributes to making hair shinier and softer as well. Olive oil acts as a natural conditioner and delivers moisture to the scalp as well as hair strands.

In addition to moisturizing agents, olive oil contains antibacterial properties that help fight common skin conditions, such as lice and dandruff, that also impact the quality of hair.

While all olive oils produce benefits for hair, extra virgin olive oil is the least processed and the purest form of olive oil

Regardless of whether to use olive oil as a dietary supplement or topical treatment to stimulate hair growth, people should use certain types of olive oils, which are high-quality extra virgin olive oils, to make hair the strongest and healthiest that it can be.

How to Use Olive Oil In Hair

The health benefits of olive oil have been proclaimed for centuries. In fact, olive oil is gaining increasing popularity as an all-natural beauty product. What it does for your body on the inside as a nutritional product, it does for your body on the outside as a beauty aid. When using olive oil in the hair, it adds moisture to both your hair follicles and your tresses. The process of using olive oil in the hair is simple, but the benefits are rewarding.

Step 1

Pour 1/2 cup of olive oil into a microwave-safe bowl. Heat it in the microwave for 20 seconds or until warm.

Step 2

Place a towel over your shoulders to protect your clothing.

Step 3

Put a small amount of olive oil in the palm of your hand and massage it into your hair. If you have a dry scalp, massage a small amount into your roots, as well. Repeat the process of massaging small amounts at a time into the hair until the hair is entirely covered with olive oil.

Step 4

Place your hair loosely on your head and cover it with a plastic shower cap.

Step 5

Relax for at least 30 minutes while the olive oil is treating your hair.

Step 6

Shampoo the olive oil out of your hair with a mild shampoo. Condition your hair with your usual conditioner to re-hydrate strands. Rinse it out completely. You will see that the olive oil treatment makes your hair much softer and much more manageable, as well as gives it some added shine.

CHAPTER 10.
HOW TO TAKE YOUR EXTRA VIRGIN OLIVE OIL

Whether you are an avid follower of The Mediterranean Diet or not, you may have heard the news that a shot of olive oil a day can keep the doctor away. Is it a myth, or is there hard evidence proving that two tablespoons of olive oil a day can reduce the risk of various life-threatening conditions, including heart disease and high LDL cholesterol?

Mostly everyone who has ever read about a diet or has looked up healthy food recipes is familiar with extra virgin olive oil, one of the best sources of monounsaturated fatty acids around. But the benefits of extra virgin olive oil like Morocco Gold are much more than just protecting the heart from disease risk. The demand for high-quality extra virgin olive oil has increased in the last few years, thanks to growth in the health-conscious populace of the world.

But did you know that drinking a shot of extra virgin olive oil first thing in the morning has a lot of health benefits too? Don't just take our word for it – here's the science!

Why Two Tablespoons of Olive Oil A Day Is Good For You

The level of polyphenols present in Morocco Gold varies slightly from year to year, depending on a range of factors, weather, time of harvesting and processing, etc. This year we are pleased to say the level of polyphenols is the highest we have yet seen.

European Food Safety Authority Recommendation

The European Food Safety Authority regulation (118) states that extra virgin olive oil with a polyphenol level of 250 mg/kg and above can make health claims. However, it is also very specific about which polyphenols this applies to. It specifically states that this must include hydroxytyrosol and its derivatives, oleuropein and tyrosol. So long as these polyphenols are present, the beneficial effects can be obtained with a daily intake of around 20ml of olive oil.

At this level of polyphenol, 1 tablespoon will have around 7.1 mg/kg (250 / 35). So, to get the health benefits, you would need to take around 3 tablespoons per day.

Due to the numerous health benefits of extra virgin olive oil, it is typically used in cooking, but eating or drinking it raw is even healthier. A lot of health experts recommend drinking extra virgin olive oil in the morning, here's why:

Benefits Of Drinking Olive Oil In The Morning

A healthy and nutritious breakfast, like a plant-based or Mediterranean diet, can help increase your chances of living a long and healthy life, according to a recent article from wellandgood.com

Based on the findings of author Dan Buettner, whose pioneering research on longevity hotspots or 'blue zones' lifts the lid on how we can potentially extend our life quality and duration, the article recommends a breakfast of foods that reduce blood pressure and cholesterol as one of 4 key choices.

The Mediterranean diet, which includes an emphasis on healthy 'monounsaturated fats' found in foods such as extra virgin olive oil, is known to help prevent a wide range of diseases such as cardiovascular disease or stroke.

Also listed in the article, entitled 4 Morning Habits of the Longest-Living People in the World, are:

Finding your 'ikigai' (the Japanese concept of what drives you to get up and out of bed in the morning).

Enjoying, a cup of morning coffee – ideally with a plant-based milk alternative and natural sweetener.

Say something nice to the first person you see. Self-explanatory this one, but Buettner starts each morning by literally complimenting others.

A shot of olive oil in the morning

If you like the sound of Buettner's teachings and want to incorporate a Mediterranean start to your day, one of the best ways to do so is by drinking a shot of extra virgin olive oil first thing in the morning. This is a quick and easy way to boost your daily intake of antioxidants and healthy fats.

You Can Also Take Extra Virgin Olive Oil Before Going To Bed

Sleep deprivation is when you don't get the sleep you need, and it is estimated to affect around one-third of American adults, a problem that has only worsened in recent years. On a society-wide level, the impacts of sleep deprivation are enormous. The CDC estimates that as many as 6,000 deaths each year are caused by drowsy driving, and sleep deprivation has been calculated to incur hundreds of billions in added healthcare costs as well as over $400B in productivity losses per year in the United States alone.

Lack of sleep directly affects how we think and feel. While the short-term impacts are more noticeable, chronic sleep deprivation can heighten the long-term risk of physical and mental health problems. To avoid these problems, it's important to avoid sleep deprivation.

What Is Sleep Deprivation?

The term sleep deprivation refers to getting less than the needed amount of sleep, which, for adults, ranges from seven to nine hours of sleep per night. Children and teens need even more nightly sleep than adults.

Different Types of Sleep Deprivation

Sleep deprivation and sleep insufficiency may be categorized in different ways depending on a person's circumstances.

Acute sleep deprivation refers to a short period, usually a few days or less, when a person has a significant reduction in their sleep time.

Chronic sleep deprivation, also known as insufficient sleep syndrome, is defined by the American Academy of Sleep Medicine (119) as curtailed sleep that persists for three months or longer.

Chronic sleep deficiency or insufficient sleep can describe ongoing sleep deprivation as well as poor sleep that occurs because of sleep fragmentation or other disruptions.

Is Sleep Deprivation Different From Insomnia?

While both insomnia and sleep deprivation involves failing to get enough sleep, many experts in sleep science make a distinction between them. People with insomnia have trouble sleeping even when they have plenty of time to sleep. On the other hand, some people with sleep deprivation don't have enough time allocated for sleep because of behaviour choices or everyday obligations.

An illustration of this difference is that people who are sleep deprived because of a busy work schedule usually have no problems sleeping longer on weekends to try to "catch up" on sleep. Someone with insomnia, however, still struggles to sleep despite having the opportunity to do so.

Multiple factors can cause or contribute to sleep deprivation, including poor sleep hygiene, lifestyle choices, work obligations, sleep disorders, and other medical conditions.

Sleep deprivation is often driven by voluntary choices that reduce available sleep time. For example, a person who decides to stay up late to binge-watch a TV series may experience acute sleep deprivation. An inconsistent sleep schedule may facilitate these decisions and make them feel less intentional at the moment.

Work obligations are another common contributor to sleep deprivation. People who work multiple jobs or extended hours may not have enough time for sufficient sleep. Shift workers who must work through the night may also find it hard to get the amount of sleep that they really need.

Sleep deficiency may be caused by other sleep disorders or medical conditions. For example, sleep apnea, a breathing disorder that induces dozens of nightly awakenings, may hinder both sleep duration and quality. Other medical or mental health problems, such as pain or general anxiety disorder, can interfere with the quality and quantity of sleep.

What Are the Symptoms of Sleep Deprivation?

The primary signs and symptoms of sleep deprivation include excessive daytime sleepiness and daytime impairment such as reduced concentration, slower thinking, and mood changes.

Feeling extremely tired during the day is one of the hallmark signs of sleep deprivation. People with excessive daytime sleepiness may feel drowsy and have a hard time staying awake even when they need to. In some cases, this results in microsleeps in which a person dozes off for a matter of seconds.

Insufficient sleep can directly affect how a person feels during their waking hours. Examples of these symptoms include:

Slowed thinking

Reduced attention span

Worsened memory

Poor or risky decision-making

Lack of energy

Mood changes - including feelings of stress, anxiety, or irritability

A person's symptoms can depend on the extent of their sleep deprivation and whether it is acute or chronic. Research also suggests that some individuals are more likely to experience symptoms after a lack of sleep and that this may be tied to a person's genetics. Stimulants like caffeine can also mask the symptoms of sleep deprivation, so it's important to note how you feel on and off these substances.

What Are the Consequences of Sleep Deprivation?

The effects of sleep deprivation and sleep deficiency (120) can be serious and far-reaching. Acute sleep deprivation raises the risk of unintentional errors and accidents. Drowsy driving, which involves slowed reaction time and the risk of microsleeps, can be life-threatening. People who are sleep-deprived are more likely to struggle in school and work settings or to experience mood changes that may affect personal relationships.

Chronic sleep deprivation can contribute to a wide range of health problems. Sleep plays a fundamental role in the effective functioning of nearly all systems of the body, so a persistent lack of sleep creates significant risks to physical and mental health:

Cardiovascular disease: Studies have found strong associations between sleep deficiency and cardiovascular problems, including high blood pressure, coronary heart disease, heart attack, and stroke.

Diabetes: Insufficient sleep appears to affect the body's ability to regulate blood sugar, increasing the risk of metabolic conditions like diabetes.

Obesity: Research has found that people tend to consume more calories and carbohydrates when they don't get enough sleep, which is just one of several ways that poor sleep may be tied to obesity and problems maintaining a healthy weight.

Immunodeficiency: Sleep deficiency has been shown to lead to worsened immune function, including a poorer response to vaccines.

Hormonal abnormalities: Sleep helps the body properly produce and regulate levels of various hormones, potentially increasing susceptibility to hormonal problems in people with sleep deprivation.

Pain: Sleep-deprived people are at a higher risk of developing pain or feeling that their pain is getting worse. Pain may cause further sleep interruptions, creating a negative cycle of worsening pain and sleep.

Mental health disorders: Sleep and mental health are closely intertwined, and poor sleep has strong associations with conditions like depression, anxiety, and bipolar disorder.

Given these diverse and important impacts of sleep deprivation, it comes as no surprise that studies have found insufficient sleep to be tied with a greater overall risk of death as well as a lower quality of life. However, all these chronic conditions can be alleviated by regular use of high-quality extra virgin olive oil like Morocco Gold.

Taking Extra Virgin Olive Oil At Bedtime: The Health Benefits

Those who suffer from sleep deprivation may benefit from the following medicinal qualities in a high-quality extra virgin olive oil. What can 2-3 tablespoons of olive oil do to get rid of insomnia?

Olive oil can help you fall asleep and sleep better in one of a few ways. First, a high-quality extra virgin olive oil can help you relax by reducing everyday inflammation that could be a potential cause for excitement.

If you work all day or even just work out in a fitness complex often, you may be experiencing some form of inflammation. Inflammation is a major cause of increased heart rate. A high-quality extra virgin olive oil can reduce the effects of inflammation, thereby calming the pace of the heart.

Pre-sleep extra virgin olive oil treatment is being suggested to those with insomnia who would like to be able to fall asleep as well as improve the quality of the given rest throughout the night. The anti-inflammatory health benefit is possible once good olive oil is taken consistently before retiring at night. Unlike some kinds of vitamins, this anti-inflammatory effect of the olive oil will not at all take long to commence functionality and promote sleep health realignment.

Secondly, extra virgin olive oil helps as a natural remedy by bringing balance to blood sugar levels that are above the average. With a high blood sugar count being a form of vasoconstriction and heart rate excitation, olive oil helping resolve this challenge is a major player in helping one fall asleep and stay asleep for a healthy amount of time.

Thirdly, the polyphenols in a high-quality extra virgin olive oil as a sleep remedy help remove a nasty molecule in your body called free radicals that can ricochet around inside your body and harm good cells. Polyphenols are a potent antioxidant, one that can work to neutralize free radicals, protecting the body from their harmful effects whilst you sleep.

Taking olive oil at bedtime can in fact, help induce relaxation as it cleanses the body of free radicals. This calming characteristic takes effect immediately. The process of ridding the body of free radicals is tiring, so, in essence, the natural consumption of a high-quality extra virgin olive oil can help you feel tired and calm.

Cooking With Extra Virgin Olive Oil

To understand the potential of extra virgin olive oil as a core ingredient in a rich and varied diet, we need to look no further than kitchens and traditions of the Mediterranean. With its emphasis on vegetables, whole grains, and healthy oils like extra virgin olive oil, The Mediterranean Diet has reached something of celebrity status across the world for decades now. But just how can I incorporate a high-quality extra virgin olive oil into my own cooking habits?

Can You Cook with Extra Virgin Olive Oil?

Possibly one of the most basic questions to start with, and the answer is a simple YES! Morocco Gold extra virgin olive oil is incredibly versatile to have on its own also as an excellent cooking medium and a flavouring ingredient. It is becoming more and more popular as a dressing for salads and pasta, for finishing cooked dishes, and for dipping with bread and raw vegetables before the meal.

High-quality extra virgin olive oils like Morocco Gold are also fine wines. They are the product of the type of olive, the soil conditions in which the olives grow, the climate, and the time the olives are harvested and pressed. This means there is a whole range of flavour profiles.

It's so versatile that you can use it in both savoury and sweet dishes, so why don't you try baking with it, as well as cooking? It's a healthier option than butter, so if that's a concern for you try it instead in your homemade cakes and biscuits, and see what you think.

The characteristics of Morocco Gold Extra Virgin Olive Oil, with its distinctive green fruitiness, hints of almond and herbs, fresh turf, and the peppery aftertaste, give a vibrant, well-balanced finish. This means using our olive oil is easy as it can be used in a variety of ways. Here are just a few uses.

Extra Virgin Olive Oil On Salads

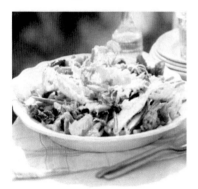

A splash of Morocco Gold extra virgin olive oil mixed with vinaigrette makes salads super healthy and taste delicious. Taking care of the microbes in our guts is one of the best ways to keep our digestive system working well and protect our immune system.

Extra Virgin Olive Oil Is Perfect As A Simple Dip

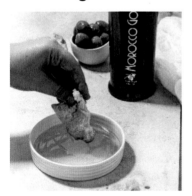

Have friends over, or fancy an evening dining Al Fresco? Using extra virgin olive oil like Morocco Gold as a dip for crispy, fresh bread is a great way to get the taste buds going. Using extra virgin olive oil like Morocco Gold as a dip for crispy, fresh bread is a great way to get the taste buds going.

Extra Virgin Olive Oil With Soups

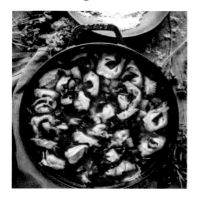

We all have our favourite go-to soup recipe. But did you know that a simple drizzle of extra virgin olive oil over your soup can make all the difference? You don't need much to seek the benefits. It adds a certain 'je ne said quoi' to the hot soup and a special richness.

Roasting with Extra Virgin Olive Oil

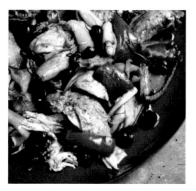

Not only does Morocco Gold extra virgin olive oil help food to cook it also adds a premium, tasty addition to the dish. High-quality extra virgin olive oil also has the unique ability to draw out and accentuate the taste of whatever you are preparing.

Pouring Extra Virgin Olive Oil Over Hot Food

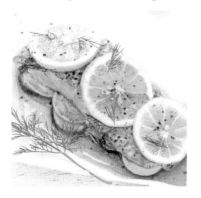

Remember that heat brings out the flavour of extra virgin olive oil, and so it will smell stronger when it is poured over hot food, and its specific flavour characteristics will be more pronounced.

Extra Virgin Olive Oil With Ice Cream

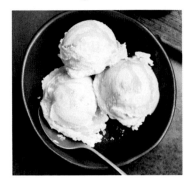

A drizzle of extra virgin olive oil over your ice cream really helps bring out the flavour in the ice cream and adds to the creamy texture. One to try out for sure! Who'd have thought it!

Why Is Extra Virgin Olive Oil Great For Cakes?

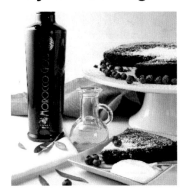

When it comes to baking, most of us assume we need certain staple ingredients, including flour, eggs, and butter. However, more and more recipes are emerging that use good-quality instead, resulting in super moist and absolutely delicious cakes.

Here's why many of us are swapping butter for olive oil in our favourite bakes and why you might too.

Extra Virgin Olive Oil Is Healthier

One of the reasons why people might prefer baking with extra virgin olive oil is because it is more nutritious than butter, which is high in saturated fat.

In comparison, extra virgin olive oil is high in mono-saturated fat, which includes antioxidants to protect our cells and vitamin E. Therefore, it is a healthier choice, as it has been shown to ease inflammation and lower the risk of developing heart disease.

Baking with it also reduces the amount of saturated fat you would otherwise consume, which raises cholesterol levels.

While you might think something bland or mild would be better in a cake or biscuit, having a strong flavour actually works in olive oil's favour when it comes to baking.

This is because it can actually taste delicious in baked goods, adding to, instead of distracting from, the overall flavour of the pudding.

The strength of extra virgin olive oil you choose will depend on what you are baking, with All Recipes suggesting using a mild variety for cakes, muffins, and cookies, as this will give the dessert a "fruity note without being overpowering".

However, you can go for a stronger type for rich puddings, such as brownies or flourless cakes.It is known to enhance the flavour of chocolate, nuts, spices, and fruit, so don't be afraid to substitute it when the recipe calls for melted butter.

According to Fine Cooking, its perfect match is a cake or bake that contains fruit or nuts, such as carrot cake or pumpkin bread.

"The extra virgin olive oil gives it a rich moistness and depth that enhances the warm spices and mingles perfectly with the essence of honey and the pumpkin seed topping," Ellie Kiriger wrote, adding: "It's an American favourite with a Mediterranean flair – a perfect package of taste and health."

The Best Olive Oil Gives Moistness To Your Baking

That brings us on to the next advantage of using extra virgin olive oil in baked goods – it makes them deliciously moist.

This is thought to be due to the vitamin E content found in extra virgin olive oil, which also helps to keep bakes fresher for longer. Indeed, while traditional cakes tend to go dry after a couple of days, those with olive oil typically stay squidgy far beyond this.

As olive oil cakes are known for their moistness, they lend themselves particularly well to bakes like carrot cake, orange cake, banana bread, lemon drizzle cake, and many other puddings that have a fruit or nut content.

Extra Virgin Olive Oil Is Great In Chocolate Cakes

Something that may surprise you is the relationship olive oil has with chocolate, particularly as the fat can have a slightly savoury flavour to it.

Despite this – or perhaps because of it – putting olive oil in chocolate cake recipes works brilliantly, giving it a rich flavour and moist texture that is difficult to replicate with butter.

As a result, there are a plethora of chocolate olive oil cake recipes available these days, including one from cookbook author and TV star Nigella Lawson.

In Nigellisima, (121) she wrote: "Although I first came up with this recipe because I had someone coming for supper who genuinely couldn't eat wheat or dairy, it is so meltingly good, I now make it all the time for those whose life and diet are not so unfairly constrained, myself included."

The cake calls for ground almonds, vanilla extract, bicarbonate of soda, caster sugar, and eggs, as well as cocoa powder and olive oil. She recommends accompanying this delicious-sounding bake with raspberries as well as mascarpone or ice cream.

A great advantage of eating a chocolate cake made with extra virgin olive oil, in addition to the flavour, is that a study has shown the combination of dark chocolate and extra virgin olive oil could improve heart health.

Research from the University of Pisa, published in Science Daily (122), revealed the two ingredients could reduce the risk of developing any cardiovascular conditions when eaten together. Dr. Rossella Di Stefano, who led the study, said: "We found that small daily portions of dark chocolate with added natural polyphenols from extra virgin olive oil was associated with an improved cardiovascular risk profile."

Extra Virgin Olive Oil Is Vegan Friendly

Another great incentive to swap butter for olive oil is that you can make your favourite puddings vegan by removing the dairy content and swapping eggs for another ingredient.

It is also a good option for those with a dairy intolerance, allowing your loved ones to continue to enjoy delicious treats without suffering an adverse reaction to it.

World's Oldest People List Olive Oil In Top Seven Foods For Long Life

The antioxidant properties and healthy (unsaturated) fats present in extra virgin olive oil make it one of the top seven foods for long life, according to some of the world's oldest people.

A recent Express.co.uk article (123) cites extra virgin olive oil and the Mediterranean Diet as one of the most trusted nutritional choices of people who enjoy a long life. The report refers to Jeanne Calment, who died in 1997 at the age of 122, and credited olive oil, port, and chocolate as the secrets to living longer.

Contributing to the article, dietitian Jenaed Brodell from Nutrition and Co (124) said: "It seems Jeanne's diet consisted of what we know as a Mediterranean eating pattern. Olive oil is the main source of fat in the Mediterranean diet.

Why Should Olive Oil Be A Staple In My Diet To Live Long?

So, just why is olive oil an important part of the Mediterranean Diet for increasing longevity? Is it all about replacing saturated fat with unsaturated fat and monounsaturated fatty acids? Protecting your heart from disease is a great way to help you live longer, but olive oil is also packed full of healthy antioxidants, which can reduce inflammation and fight off a range of diseases.

Brodell explains, "Olive oil is high in healthy fats as well as having great antioxidant properties. People who consume this diet appear to have a higher life expectancy, including a lower chance of dying from cardiovascular diseases."

The World's Healthiest Village

There are numerous studies that point to the health benefits of extra virgin olive oil like Morocco Gold.

Pioppi, Italy, is known as the world's healthiest village (125) because many of its residents live past the age of 100. The villagers have a diet of whole natural foods comprised of things that are in season and available according to the local climate.

Imagine living in a community where the average man lives to be 89, and many reach the 100-year mark. Picture what it would be like to enjoy one's golden years without dementia or type 2 diabetes, maladies that are an integral part of aging in the rest of the world. After hearing about Pioppi, cardiologist Aseem Malhotra became fascinated with discovering what diet kept the residents so healthy and what lessons could be learned from them.

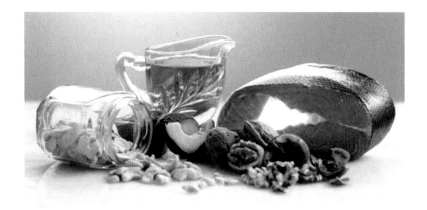

After studying the village, Malhotra developed a formula for optimal health. For starters, the Pioppians have a very low sugar intake, eating it only once per week. It is this dietary practice that the doctor considers essential for their good health. He contends that western society's fear of fat is to blame for the high consumption of sugar and refined carbohydrates. Malhotra attributes these foods as the cause of the widespread incidence of heart disease, type 2 diabetes, and obesity.

Pioppi has received notoriety because it's known as the home of the Mediterranean diet. As the villagers have no supermarket, their diet consists largely of vegetables, olive oil, and fish. They also eat cheese, but other dairy products aren't available. Pasta and bread are consumed in small quantities. In addition to sugar, their diet is low in meat and refined carbohydrates.

Other lifestyle practices aside from a healthful diet play a role. The villagers get seven hours of sleep per night and experience freedom from much stress. Although it isn't intentional, intermittent fasting is a natural part of their lives. They don't engage in exercise per se, but they're very active.

Included in his top recommendations for vibrant health and longevity based on the Pioppians:

Extra virgin olive oil is medicine – take it every day.

One further consideration – who would not want to live forever in a place like this!!

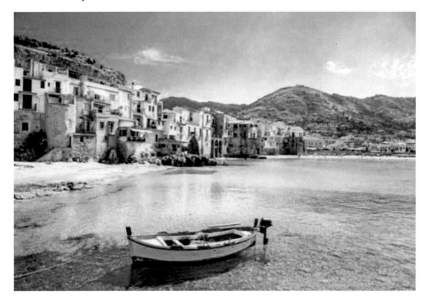

REFERENCES

1) 150,000 Litres of Fraudulent Oil Seized by Europol. Europol headquarters in The Hague May 21, 2019.

2) The Telegraph: 'Fake' olive oil is making its way to the UK, experts warn 10 September 2017

3) Olive-oil industry model "broken", warns Deoleo CEO 13 July 2018

4) Forbes: Sir, Perhaps Some Perrier In Your Benzene? Apr 23, 2019

5) Scientific Opinion on the substantiation of a health claim related to polyphenols in olive and maintenance of normal blood HDL cholesterol concentrations (ID 1639, further assessment) pursuant to Article 13(1) of Regulation (EC) No 1924/2006 Published:7 August 2012 Adopted: 28 June 2012

6) New Insights Into the World's Oldest Bottle of Olive Oil. University of Naples Federico II department of agriscience (DIA). Nov. 29, 2020

7) New insights into Early Celtic consumption practices: Organic residue analyses of local and imported pottery from Vix-Mont Lassois. June 2019 Philipp Stockhammer.

8) Nancy Ash, The Olive Source
9) Mat's World, The Olive Oil Source

10) The Telegraph: British supermarkets admit their olive oils could be killing birds as they pledge to switch brands. 29 MAY 2019

11) Michael A Clark, Marco Springmann, Jason Hill, and David Tilman, published in the journal Proceedings of the National Academy of Sciences (PNAS)

12) Paolo Amirante, Alistair G. Paice, Olives and Olive Oil in Health and Disease Prevention, 2010

13) Anti-Inflammatory Effect of 3,4-DHPEA-EDA www.researchgate.net › publication › 225288529

14) Biological Relevance of Extra Virgin Olive Oil Polyphenols Metabolites. Department of Biomedical Sciences, University of Cagliari, Cittadella Universitaria, Monserrato, Italy. Published: 22 November 2018

15) Identification of lignans as major components in the phenolic fraction of olive oil - PubMed (nih.gov)

16) Spanish scientists confirm extra virgin olive oil helps to combat breast cancer

17) Faculty Of Pharmacy Seville and the Biomedical Research Institute Coruna (M.S. Meiss, M. Sanchez-Hidalgo, A. González-Benjumea)

18) Osteoarthritis treatment with a novel nutraceutical acetylated ... journals.sagepub.com › doi › abs

19) Oleuropein aglycone: A polyphenol with different targets.
www.sciencedirect.com › science › article › pii

20) Structure Properties, Acquisition Protocols, Frontiers.
www.frontiersin.org › articles › fchem.2018.00239

21) Dr Limor Goren PhD, City University of New York.

22) Tyrosol an overview Science Direct Topics
www.sciencedirect.com › topics › medicine-and-dentistry

23) Michael A Clark, Marco Springmann, Jason Hill, and David
Tilman, published in the journal Proceedings of the
National Academy of Sciences (PNAS)

24) Cardiovascular diseases (CVDs) World Health
Organization

25) Cardiovascular Disease - Health Metrics - American Heart

26) Suffering in Silence: The Hidden Costs of Digestive
Disease Stigma for Employers

27) Trends in Healthcare Expenditures Among US Adults With
Hypertension: National Estimates, 2003–2014

28) New figures show high blood pressure costs NHS billions
each year, NHS England

29) Effects of Olive Oil on Blood Pressure: Epidemiological,
Clinical, and Mechanistic Evidence, Marika
Massaro, Egeria Scoditti, Maria Annunziata Carluccio,

Nadia Calabriso, Giuseppe Santarpino, Tiziano Verri, and Raffaele De Caterina. Published online 2020 May 26.

30) www.pfizer.com › news › featured_stories_detail › chr...

31) www.verywellhealth.com/signs-of-inflammation-4580526

32) www.health.harvard.edu/staying-healthy/foods-that-fight-inflammation

33) Structure Properties, Acquisition Protocols, and ww.frontiersin.org>articles>fchem.2018.00239>full

34) High Cholesterol Facts | cdc.gov

35) The Lancet: The Lyon Diet Heart Study

36) Published online 2015 Jul 26. doi: 10.4330/wjc.v7.i7.404

37) American Heart Association's journal *Circulation.* Cardiovascular Risk and Nutrition Research Group at the Hospital del Mar Medical Research Institute in Barcelona, Spain.

38) www.medicalnewstoday.com/articles/315818.php?bl

39) Exploitation Of Recent Breakthroughs - Brown and Goldstein – 1996

40) Published online 2015 Jul 26. doi: 10.4330/wjc.v7.i7.404

41) The Cost of Diabetes | ADA - American Diabetes Association www.diabetes.org › resources › statistics › cost-diabetes

42) The costs of drug prescriptions for diabetes in the NHS - www.thelancet.com › PIIS0140-6736(18)33190-8 ›

43) National Library Of Medicine Olive oil has a beneficial effect on impaired glucose regulation and other cardiometabolic risk factors. Di@bet.es study, 2013 Jul 17

44) Sapienza University in Romen

45) Extra virgin olive oil lowers blood glucose and cholesterol

46) www.diabetes.co.uk › news › sep › extra-virgin-olive-oil-

47) https://www.beatoapp.com/blog/how-do-i-lower-my-blood-glucose-levels/

48) Trends in Healthcare Expenditures Among US Adults With Hypertension: National Estimates, 2003–2014

49) New figures show high blood pressure costs NHS billions each year, NHS England

50) Olive oil and reduced need for antihypertensive medications, L A Ferrara [1], A S Raimondi, L d'Episcopo, L Guida, A Dello Russo, T Marotta, 2000 Mar

51) Medical costs of osteoporosis in the elderly Medicare population. S W Blume, J R Curtis MID: 21165602

52) European Prospective Investigation into Cancer and
    Nutrition Study

53) https://www.oastaug.com/orthopaedic-specialties/spine-
    center/osteoporosis/

54) osteoporosis among the elderly.26 Jul 2016
    Olives and Bone: A Green Osteoporosis Prevention Option

55) Epidemiology of Osteoarthritis, Yuqing Zhang,
    D.Sc and Joanne M. Jordan, MD, MPH, 2010 Aug; 26(3):
    355–369.

56) Faculty Of Pharmacy Seville and the Biomedical Research
    Institute Coruna (M.S. Meiss, M. Sanchez-Hidalgo, A.
    González-Benjumea)

57) Osteoarthritis treatment with a novel nutraceutical
    acetylated journals.sagepub.com › doi › abs

58) Filomena Nazaro, senior scientist at the National Research
    Council's Institute of Food Sciences, Italy

59) Dr Limor Goren, Hunter College of the City University of
    New York, and Dr David Foster,

60) Weill Cornell Medicine, Rutgers University, and Albert
    Einstein College of Medicine
61) Dr Javier Menendez Catalan Institute of Oncology in Spain

62) Journal of Nutritional Biochemistry, 2016,

63) Nutrition & Metabolism, 2015

64) Harvard School of Public Health: Nutrition and Immunity

65) The Journal of the American Medical Association Cara Ebbeling PhD, and David Ludwig, MD, of the New Balance Foundation Obesity Prevention Center at Boston Children's Hospital,

66) Runners World, Lori Russell

67) Short-Term Mediterranean Diet Improves Endurance Exercise Performance: A Randomized-Sequence Crossover Trial

68) 2021 study in the International Journal of Obesity.

69) Jesús de la Osada, Professor of Biochemistry at the Faculty of Veterinary Medicine of the University of Zaragoza.

70) 5 Ways to Sweeten Your Sex Life With A Little Olive Oil Lubricant https://www.honeycolony.com › ... › Love & Sex

71) University of Athens

72) Julie Ward, Senior Cardiac Nurse at the British Heart Foundation

73) Dr Clive Petry, Benefits of EVOO for couples who are trying to conceive https://olivewellnessinstitute.org › Articles

74) Dr.Associations between dietary patterns and semen quality in men undergoing IVF/ICSI treatment June 2009

75) Association between adherence to the Mediterranean diet and semen quality parameters in male partners of couples_attempting_fertility,_Dimitrios_Karayiannis, Meropi D. Kontogianni, Christina Mendorou, Lygeri Douka, Minas Mastrominas, Nikos Yiannakouris, January 2017.

76) Harvard T.H. Chan School of Public Health

77) Nurses' Health Study (NHS)

78) Health Professionals Follow-up Study (HPFS)

79) https://www.health.harvard.edu/blog/healthy-lifestyle-5-keys-to-a-longer-life-2018070514186

80) University of Navarra and Las Palmas de Gran Canaria,

81) Dr Drew Ramsey, M.D. Professor of psychiatry at Columbia University, April 2018,

82) The 'SMILES' trial Australia

83) Naturopathic Physician Vickie Modica of Seattle, Washington

84) Aristotle University of Thessaloniki and the Greek Association of Alzheimer's Disease and Related Disorders – Journal Of Alzheimer's Disease

85) Tommaso Ballarini, Ph.D. The American Academy of Neurology

86) Kristin Kirkpatrick, Cleveland Clinic - Medical News Today

87) Dr Richard Isaacson, Alzheimer's Prevention Clinic at Weill Cornell Medicine and New York Presbyterian Hospital

88) National Herald

89) News Medical

90) Lewis Katz School of Medicine, Temple University, Philadelphia

91) http://www.sciencetimes.com/articles/17281/20170625/extr a-virgin-olive-oil-discovered-preserve-memory-prevent-alzheimer-s.htm

92) Oleuropein aglycone: A polyphenol with different targets www.sciencedirect.com › science › article ›

93) Khalid El Sayed, Professor Of Pharmaceutical and Toxicological Sciences, University of Louisiana-Monroe

94) "MIND" Diet, Mediterranean-DASH (Dietary Approaches to Stop Hypertension) Intervention for Neurodegenerative Delay. International Parkinson and Movement Disorder Society.

95) Silke Appel-Cresswell, Neurologist, University Of British Columbia, Faculty of Medicine

96) Neurology, Megu Baden, PhD, Department of Nutrition at the Harvard T.H. Chan School of Public Health

97) Medscape Erica Camargo Faye, MD, PhD, Massachusetts General Hospital & Harvard Medical School, Boston, Massachusetts:

98) Neurology®, Cécilia Samieri, PhD, University of Bordeaux and the National Institute of Health and Medical Research

99) PLoS ONE. Charles Hong, MD, PhD, Professor of medicine and director of cardiology research at the University of Maryland School of Medicine.

100)   New risk factors linked to increased risk of COVID-19 infection https://www.eurekalert.org › news-releases

101)   Lancet. COVID-19: consider cytokine storm syndromes and immunosuppression. Puja Mehta, Daniel F McAuley Michael Brown Emilie Sanchez, Rachel S Tattersall, Jessica J Manson, and HLH across Speciality Collaboration, UK. 2020 28 March-3 April.

102)   European Centre for Disease Prevention and Control, (Latest update 30 September 2021)

103) scientificanimations.com, CC BY-SA

104) The role of macrophages in obesity-associated islet inflammation and β-cell abnormalities, Wei Ying, Wenxian Fu, Yun Sok Lee & Jerrold M. Olefsky, Published: 13 December 2019

105) Sheena Cruickshank, Professor in Biomedical Sciences, University of Manchester The key factor that explains vulnerability to severe COVID https://www.manchester.ac.uk › discover › news › inflam...

106) European Journal of Clinical Nutrition, Dietary changes and anxiety during the coronavirus pandemic: a multinational survey, Vered Kaufman-Shriqui, Daniela Abigail Navarro, Olga Raz & Mona Boaz, Published: 19 March 2021

107) A randomised controlled trial of dietary improvement for adults with major depression (the 'SMILES' trial) Published: 30 January 2017

108) New England Journal Of Medicine, Primary Prevention of Cardiovascular Disease with a Mediterranean Diet Supplemented with Extra-Virgin Olive Oil or Nut

109) University Of Malaga, Cápsulas con aceite de oliva frente a la covid, 04/03/2021

110) The Olive Press, Andalusian hospital explores health benefits of Spain's 'liquid ...1st Mar 2021

111) Ahmad Alkhatib, Teeside University Centre For Public Health, Antiviral Functional Foods and Exercise Lifestyle Prevention of Coronavirus, 28 Aug 2020,

112) University Of Navarra, Pamplona, Mediterranean diet, and telomere length in high cardiovascular risk subjects from the PREDIMED-NAVARRA study, 2016 Apr 1.

113) National Library Of Medecine, Mediterranean Diet and Telomere Length: A Systematic Review and Meta-Analysis , Silvia Canudas, Nerea Becerra-Tomás, Pablo Hernández-Alonso, Serena Galié, Cindy Leung , Published: 30 July 2020

114) How to Use Olive Oil for Hair Care, Medically reviewed by Gerhard Whitworth, R.N. Written by Elea Carey Updated on February 26, 2019

115) Olive Oil vs. Coconut Oil: Which One Wins In The Beauty Department? Stuti Bhattacharya Updated: Jan 17, 2022, 19:44 IST

116) Elle, Shop Miranda Kerr's Beauty Closet, Justine Harman Sep 19, 2013

117) Good Housekeeping, Why You Should Use Olive Oil for Your Hair By Nicole Blades Sep 16, 2019

118) European Food Safety Authority, Scientific Opinion on the substantiation of a health claim 7 Aug 2012

119)   American Academy of Sleep Medicine

120)   Sleep Deprivation: Causes, Symptoms, & Treatment. www.sleepfoundation.org › sleep-deprivation

121)   Nigella Lawson, Chocolate Olive Oil Cake, Nigellissima

122)   European Society of Cardiology, Dark chocolate with olive oil associated with improved cardiovascular risk profile August 29, 2017

123)   The Express, How to live longer: 7 foods the world's oldest people swear by and if they'll work for you, Miranda Slade Sep 12, 2021

124)   www.nutritionandco.co.uk

125)   www.institutefornaturalhealing.com/2017/09/secrets-worlds-healthiest-village/